Cosmic Detox

Cosmic Detox

A Taoist Approach
to Internal Cleansing

Mantak Chia
and
William U. Wei

Destiny Books
Rochester, Vermont • Toronto, Canada

Destiny Books
One Park Street
Rochester, Vermont 05767
www.DestinyBooks.com

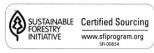

Destiny Books is a division of Inner Traditions International

Originally published in Thailand in 2009 by Universal Tao Publications under the title *Cosmic Cleansing: Internal Cleansing through the Cosmos*

Library of Congress Cataloging-in-Publication Data
Chia, Mantak, 1944–
  Cosmic detox : a taoist approach to internal cleansing / Mantak Chia and William U. Wei.
      p. cm.
  Includes index.
  ISBN 978-1-59477-377-8 (pbk.)
  1. Detoxification (Health) 2. Taoist hygiene. I. Wei, William U. II. Title.
  RA784.5.C45 2011
  613—dc22

                                                                    2011006220

Printed and bound in the United States by Lake Book Manufacturing
The text paper is SFI certified. The Sustainable Forestry Initiative® program promotes sustainable forest management.

10   9   8   7   6   5   4   3   2   1

Text design by Priscilla H. Baker
Text layout by Virginia Scott Bowman
This book was typeset in Janson Text and Futura with Present and Futura as display typefaces

Photographs by Saysunee Yongyod
Illustrations by Udon Jandee

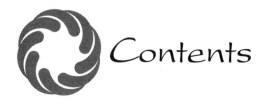

Contents

Acknowledgments

We extend our gratitude to the many generations of Taoist Masters who have passed on their special lineage, in the form of an unbroken oral transmission, over thousands of years. We thank Taoist Master I Yun (Yi Eng) for his openness in transmitting the formulas of Taoist Inner Alchemy. We also wish to thank the thousands of unknown men and women of the Chinese healing arts who developed many of the methods and ideas presented in this book.

We offer our eternal gratitude to our parents and teachers for their many gifts to us. Remembering them brings joy and satisfaction to our continued efforts in presenting the Universal Healing Tao System. For their gifts, we offer our eternal gratitude and love. As always, their contribution has been crucial in presenting the concepts and techniques of the Universal Healing Tao.

We thank the many contributors essential to this book's final form: The editorial and production staff at Inner Traditions/Destiny Books for their efforts to clarify the text and produce a handsome new edition of the book and Gail Rex for her line edit of the new edition.

We wish to thank the following people who contributed to the earlier editions of this book: Bob Zuraw for sharing his kindness, healing techniques, and Taoist understandings; Lee Holden for his editorial work and writing contributions; Colin Drown for his editorial work; Otto Thamboon for his artisic contributions; our Senior Instructors, Wilbert Wils and Saumya Wils, for their insight; and Matthew Koren, without whom the book would not have come to be; and special thanks to our Thai Production Team, Hirunyathorn Punsan, Saysunee Yongyod, Udon Jandee, and Saniem Chaisam.

Putting Cosmic Detox into Practice

The practices described in this book have been used successfully for thousands of years by Taoists trained by personal instruction. Readers should not undertake the practice without receiving personal transmission and training from a certified instructor of the Universal Healing Tao, since certain of these practices, if done improperly, may cause injury or result in health problems. This book is intended to supplement individual training by the Universal Healing Tao and to serve as a reference guide for these practices. Anyone who undertakes these practices on the basis of this book alone, does so entirely at his or her own risk.

The meditations, practices, and techniques described herein are not intended to be used as an alternative or substitute for professional medical treatment and care. If any readers are suffering from illnesses based on mental or emotional disorders, an appropriate professional health care practitioner or therapist should be consulted. Such problems should be corrected before you start training.

Neither the Universal Healing Tao nor its staff and instructors can be responsible for the consequences of any practice or misuse of the information contained in this book. If the reader undertakes any exercise without strictly following the instructions, notes, and warnings, the responsibility must lie solely with the reader.

This book does not attempt to give any medical diagnosis, treatment, prescription, or remedial recommendation in relation to any human disease, ailment, suffering or physical condition whatsoever.

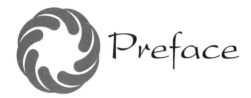 Preface

This book is about your power to heal yourself. More specifically, it addresses your body's inherent ability to heal itself by regularly cleaning out the nine openings of the body on a cellular level. It is that simple; that is the Tao. Take a moment to think about it: How would you live your life differently knowing you had access to immense levels of health and energy? How much more would you be able to do with your life? How much less would you be able to do with your life?

Although we will ostensibly be talking about physical healing, remember that what heals the physical body also heals our emotional and spiritual selves. We are talking about a transformation of being, and indeed, you will need to slough off old patterns and past behaviors to really benefit from the accumulated knowledge in this book.

The body going through life is like a river winding through a forest. As the river flows through at varying speeds and currents, blockages can occur. Branches and trees sometimes fall in, mud builds up, and animals swim through leaving waste products behind. These can eventually turn the river into a swamp. The only way to get the water flowing freely again is to clear the branches and other debris out of the way.

The same thing happens with the human body. In fact, the body has many energy rivers; blockages are created in them when imbalanced blood and mucus begin to get stuck instead of flowing freely. These stagnancies then eat away at the body in a decay process called aging. Orifices are typically the first areas to become blocked. Energy is focused through them, so anything blocking them can disrupt the flow and create widespread havoc.

Why worry about blockages and sickness? Aren't they a natural part of life? In our current culture, they are unfortunately a big part of life, though they don't need to be. Certainly your level of health is your choice, but it is important to realize that such blockages also prevent your spiritual evolution. Consciousness does not stay in a diseased body for long. It is impossible to practice meditation and movement in such a body, and you will never live long enough to evolve. Yet, it is through meditation practices that you have an opportunity to achieve longevity.

Taoists came up with the cleansing processes described in this book to keep the energy rivers free flowing; by regularly cleaning them out, we thereby clear the way for higher-level practices that encourage the body to replace old, unhealthy cells with new healthy ones.

The concept of this book is first to offer different strategies and techniques for opening up blockages within the body. Once the blockages have been removed, deeper-level cleansing and healing can take place. The material in this book is organized by the body's nine openings: the colon, the urinary tract, two eyes, two ears, two nostrils, and the mouth. We will move through the body orifice by orifice, noting the function of each opening, its associated behaviors, emotions, and related organs according to Chinese medicine, as well as noting common blockages and how to cleanse them. By the end of your journey, you will have touched all the major openings that can contribute to blockages within your body. Then we will shift gears and learn about more general cellular cleansing systems and prevention strategies. The book will end with guidelines for a fourteen-day total-body cleanse that can be practiced every six months.

In talking about ourselves, we often assume a dichotomy between "myself" and "my body." This is pure comedy. You are your body, and your body is you. If your body can heal itself, you can heal yourself. Get it? It is not that radical an idea, and you do not have to agree or disagree. There is merely what actually works and what does not work for the time and place in which you find yourself. Everyone's body is as different as their experiences. Some of the cleansing methods in this book will work for you, and some will not be as effective, depending on your condition of health. I encourage you to experiment with yourself and with your friends. Try variations, discover new ways of being, but most of all, have fun and enjoy the ride on your life's journey.

Your Friend in the Tao,
William U. Wei
Wei Tzu—The Professor—Master of Nothingness
The Myth that Takes the Mystery out of Mysticism

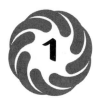

Detoxification Theory and Concepts

Taoist sages in the mountains have refined their bodies and minds to a great degree. They can absorb dew from the air, and that becomes their nourishment; they become like trees. Their bodies can recirculate water at will, and can generate enough heat in any situation so that they do not need clothing. They do not become ill. The sages can do all this because they know how to maintain their bodies in accordance with natural laws (fig. 1.1).

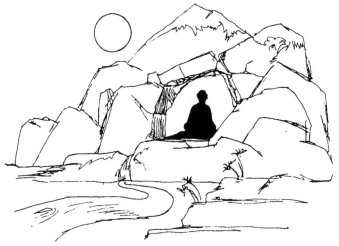

Fig.1.1. Taoist sage meditating in a mountain cave

The possibility of health, beauty, grace, truth, and wisdom that are everlastingly immune to all forms of disease is probably one of the most sought after attainments of man. To those willing to listen and give heed to the voice of Mother Nature, all of these blessings are within easy reach. Vigorous health, life-long usefulness, and a happy, carefree future are the rightful heritage of every individual, promising a happier and spiritually enlightened future, along with that greatly desired longevity. The secret is in the power of cleansing.

There are many ways to cleanse the body, and learning to do so correctly will bring you to unimagined levels of health and vitality. Conversely, if you do not learn to cleanse at all, degenerative diseases will result. In the chapters that follow, you will be introduced to detailed methods for cleansing the body, beginning with the nine openings (two eyes, two ears, two nostrils, mouth, anus, and genitals) and moving on to more general methods of cleansing at the cellular level.

Such cleanses are intended to be bimodal—cleansing to the spirit as well as to the body. This is the only way to regain right relationship with natural laws. By reacquainting ourselves with nature's fundamental teachings regarding the proper care of the human body, we can once again celebrate the foundational teachings of unity, the religion of love that is every being's birthright.

IMPROPER FOOD IS A CAUSE OF DISEASE

The earliest humans lived in an environment that provided invisible food as they roamed: perfume from trees and other vegetation; pure, clear, sparkling water that was unpolluted and free from chemical additives and poisonous gases; magnetic impulses received through contact with the clean soil; and electric vibrations communicated through the luxuriant growth of hair on the head and body (for each single hair is an electric-receiving station). Direct, life-giving rays were received from the sun on the naked skin.

These invisible foods fed both the body and spirit, which are inexorably interconnected. Compare this with our present-day food, which is frequently damaged or fake, or completely lost in processing. Even our organically grown foods do not escape the damage of depleted soils, genetic modifications, and long-distance travel.

The widespread pollution of our essential food sources leads to the many diseases and bodily ailments afflicting modern mankind—especially all kinds of degenerative diseases. It is only when we begin to eliminate these causes of illness that we will discover the experience of true good health.

It has long been recognized that certain foods are not suitable for mankind. They cannot be fully digested, so they remain in the tissues of the body as a sticky, gluey mucus that eventually clogs the entire circulation. Incompletely digestible foods may be those of poor quality—especially mucus-forming foods like fats, dairy products, meats, and starches—or simply those of too much quantity: most people eat too much, and this, too, causes a buildup of mucus. These partially digested materials cannot be properly eliminated, so they begin to decay within the digestive system. Incompletely broken down molecules enter the bloodstream and poison it, carrying diseased material to the various organs of the body.

People living on the accepted present-day "mixed" diet of meat, starches, and liquids—and even those on a starchy vegetarian regimen—have systems that are essentially clogged with mucus. But we may still have time to readjust to nature's guidelines and reinstitute the paradise of old. Man may, in fact, reacquire the enduring vitality to live for hundreds of years at full vigor, just as he did when first put on Earth. In order to do this, however, he must inevitably return to a natural diet. Health will not return, nor can it be regained, through drug remedies or other medical treatments, since supreme, absolute, heavenly health is ruled by the laws of diet. All other methods must be classified as aids and come under the category of assistance.

The more intelligent a human being becomes, the more careful he or she is about diet. The highest degree of real civilization—of mental and spiritual development—can be reached only in a most perfect body, which can only be developed by means of a pure diet, periodic cleansing, exercise, and meditation. No individual can hope to attain this much-desired state if he or she fails to properly care for his or her body in accordance with nature's methods in every respect. Whether humans experience growth from childhood to maturity—like every other living organism—or endless cycles of disease, is dependent upon the type of food they eat.

The high-protein diets and stimulant foods, such as coffee and alcohol, that are common today result in a decline of vigor in both men and women. These diets increase the metabolic rate and blood pressure, along with the production of uric acid. In men, such a diet will promote sexual excesses due to overexcitation of the genital mucosal membranes. Women will frequently be afflicted with painful menstrual cycles and problems with the genital tract and reproductive organs. Poor digestion is certainly a result of poor diets in both sexes, and the cause of weakened physical, intellectual, and spiritual capacities of all types. In contrast, an alkaline diet, which tends to be more calming and counteracts the formation of uric acid, serves to reduce intense sexual impulses and the types of intense behavior that can be socially dysfunctional as well as biologically and spiritually harmful.

It should be noted that highly stimulating diets, which reduce vitality and activity in the higher centers of the body, are very different than substances such as ginseng, which have a definite vitalizing and rejuvenating action on the sex glands.

THE IDEAL DIET

We needn't look far for a diet that does not lead to a buildup of mucus in the body: from our earliest history, mankind's most available, most natural food source was a fruit orchard. Today, a heavenly diet of fresh fruit is not only possible, but is the way to start the deep cleansing process that has become necessary for mankind. In fact, the nutritive and curative values of fresh fruits and starch-less vegetables are far superior to all other foods. They not only furnish the blood with the best nutrient elements and solvents, but starchless green vegetables (such as kale and collard greens) contain high mineral-salt contents and valuable vitamins. If man lived in accordance with natural dietetic laws, on a mucus-free diet, he would experience absolute health, beauty, and strength with no pain or grief (fig. 1.2).

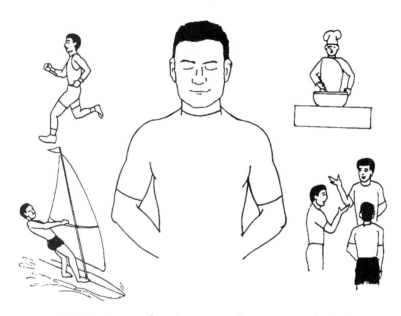

Fig.1.2. A mucus-free diet stops inflammation in the body.

However, a sudden or too rapid change from the "wrong" foods to an exclusive fruit diet often causes undesirable disturbances even in the body of a healthy individual. It is therefore preferable that the change from today's accepted diet of meat, bread, and potatoes be accomplished through following a transitional diet. A transitional diet would be based on the idea that 75–80 percent of our foods should be alkalizing to the body, and only 20–25 percent should be acidifying.

Just as an example, a long transition diet is necessary for individuals who from early childhood were given drug remedies for their various ills, whether through innocence or plain ignorance. The harmful properties contained in these drugs are ever present, and take years for complete elimination.

Alkaline versus Acid

One of the basic dynamics in the body is the relationship between acidity and alkalinity. The bloodstream's optimal pH is very slightly alkaline—measuring 7.36 on the pH scale. This slightly alkaline environment allows the body to remove toxins, repair tissues, and maintain optimal cellular function. An acid environment, on the other hand, creates toxins, prevents their efficient removal, and leads to many disease processes including fatigue, heart disease, osteoporosis, and possibly cancer as well. Whether our bodies are predominantly acid or alkaline depends largely on the foods we eat (fig. 1.3).

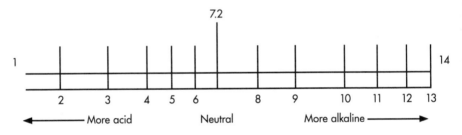

Fig. 1.3. The pH scale

Once food enters the body it is broken down and digested; what we actually assimilate then is not the physical food form itself, but the energetic form—a kind of digested resin that gives off a positive and negative charge. How we utilize that charge is really determined by the internal environment of the body. If the internal environment is not well balanced—if it is too acidic, for instance—we may react badly to the energetic charge of the foods, becoming sluggish or ill.

The key is to consciously utilize our meals to balance and fortify our internal environments. This will allow the body to perform its natural process of cleansing to remove built-up acids and other stored toxins. The way people have done this for centuries is to maintain themselves on an alkaline diet.

However, most typical diets tend to push the body into mild or even pronounced acidity. This creates a chemical imbalance in the body. The acid-producing foods in the West that would create this syndrome are animal products and a lot of foods that actually ferment in the body because of the sugar content (condiments, junk foods, candies, pastries).

The uric and sulfuric acids created by so many of the foods we eat is neutralized in the body with calcium. If your body did not neutralize these acids with calcium you would die of internal hemorrhaging from holes burned in your arteries. Instead, the body draws calcium from the bloodstream and the bones. It actually draws out the calcium—your alkaline reserves—from the bones to neutralize the uric acid in the bloodstream.

Over a period of time, say, forty or fifty years, this results in osteoporosis, which occurs in women around the age of sixty-six and in men about the age of eighty. The spine starts to bend, creating a hunched-over posture, while the bones become brittle and easily breakable. Your body literally shrinks because the calcium is being leached out of your bones to neutralize the uric acid from the consumption of animal products. To complicate matters further, all the calcium that goes into your bloodstream then gets filtered through your kidneys, which places a large burden on these vital detoxifiers. This is how we get kidney stones, gallstones, and arthritis.

Clearly, we all have an interest in avoiding these disease scenarios, yet the way to alkalinize our bodies is not always clear. Some foods might be acidic in their fresh state—like fresh grapefruit, for instance—but may actually have an alkalinizing effect on the body once they have been digested. We need to consume foods that are slightly alkaline once we have completely digested them.

Instead of protein from meat and animal products as the major part of a meal, greens become the nutritional foundation. Examples would be broccoli, collard greens, wheat greens, cucumbers, lettuces (romaine and bib), and kale. We also eat grasses, root vegetables—such as onions, radishes, daikon, carrots, turnips, sweet potatoes, yams, and beets—and sprouted whole grains (fig. 1.4).

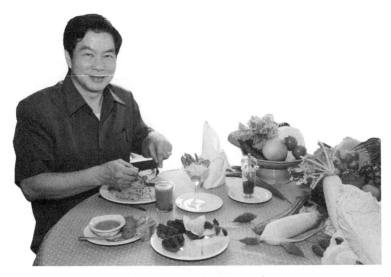

Fig. 1.4. An alkaline meal

By eating a diet like this that is 80 percent alkaline and 20 percent acidic, you would eliminate any allergies, skin problems, digestive troubles, and many chronic conditions. Fatigue would become a thing of the past, because the energy in your body would return to a natural state of flow.

The sections below detail some common foods and their effects on our acid/alkaline balance. Keep in mind, however, that there is some disagreement among various sources about whether particular foods are acidifying or alkalizing, so you may find what appear to be contradictions between this material and other sources on this subject.

Alkaline-Forming Foods

The following foods are considered to be alkalizing in the body when eaten fresh or lightly steamed.

Fresh Vegetables

Artichokes, asparagus, avocados, bamboo shoots, beans (string, wax, lima, and soy), beets, cabbage (red), carrots, celery, chard, chives, corn, cucumbers, endive, garlic, herbs (all), horseradish, kale, kohl-rabi, leeks, lettuce (leaf), okra, onions (some), parsley, parsnips, peas (fresh), peppers (sweet), pimento, potatoes (red and sweet), pumpkin, rutabagas, sauerkraut, spinach (raw), sprouts (all), squash (summer), tomatoes (yellow), watercress, yams

Fresh Fruits

Apples (golden delicious), apricots (very ripe), berries (except blueberries), cherries (bing), grapefruit (pink), grapes, kumquats, lemons (tree ripened), mango, longan berries, loquats, melons (all kinds), papaya, passion fruit

Nuts (Raw and Soaked)

Almonds, macadamias, pecans

Starches and Sugars

Carob, cornbread (yellow), cornmeal (yellow), cornmeal cereal, cornstarch crackers (alkaline/whole-grains), hominy, spaghetti (egg noodle), popcorn (yellow), maple syrup (100 percent pure), pancakes (alkaline flour), pastries (alkaline flour), peas (dried green), brown rice (short grain), vegetable pasta

Flours

Artichoke flour, cornmeal, durum flour, oat flour, rye flour

Proteins

Avocados (ripe), dried beans (lima, pinto), buttermilk, clams, cheese (white), cow's milk (raw), cornish hen, duck, fish (lean, such as sole, trout, perch), goat milk (raw), lamb, nuts, rabbit, seeds (all when sprouted), soy milk, soybean sprouts, turtle, yogurt (plain)

Miscellaneous

Butter (sweet), chlorophyll, herbal teas, olive oil

Acid-Forming Foods

The following foods are considered to be acid-forming in the system.

Fresh Vegetables

Brussels sprouts, broccoli, cauliflower, cabbage,* eggplant, lettuce (iceberg), mushroom, radishes, tomatoes (red)

Fresh Fruits

Apple (red and green), blueberries, cherries (light), currants, cranberries, dates, figs, grapefruit (white), nectarines, olives, oranges, peaches (most), pears (bartlett), persimmons, pineapple, plums, prunes, pomegranate, raspberries, rhubarb, quince, strawberries (tart), tangerines

Nuts (Raw)

Hickory, pine, pistachio, walnuts (black and English)

Starches and Sugars

Banana squash, barley, bran, bread (graham, rye, white, whole wheat), cereals (all kinds, packaged), cornmeal (white), crackers (white), doughnuts, dressings, dry beans (most), dumplings (white), flour (list), gravies (most kinds), honey, hubbard squash, jelly (all kinds), jerusalem artichokes, molasses, pancakes (white), pastries (white), peanuts, peas (dried white, yellow), potatoes (brown skin), preserves (white sugar), puddings, pumpkin, rice (white/wild/long-grain brown), rye, soups (thick), spaghetti (white), sugar (all kinds), syrups (white sugar), tapioca, waffles (white), wheat

---

*The cruciferous vegetables (broccoli, brussels sprouts, cabbage, etc.) contain sulfur, which is itself acid, but they can also restore minerals to a person suffering from acidification. Only those who are overly sensitive to acids need exclude them from the diet. Others may eat them in moderation to healthful effect.

Flours

Brown rice, buckwheat, barley, gluten, whole wheat, soy

Proteins

Cashews, catfish, cheese (yellow), crabs, eggs, fish (pink), hazel nuts, hickory nuts, lentils, lobster, meats (beef/pork/veal), mutton, olives (green), oysters, peanut (legume), peanut butter, pine nuts, pistachio nuts, poultry (chicken), turkey (dark meat), shrimp, scallops, squab, venison (wild), milk (low protein)

Miscellaneous

Canned and prepared foods tend toward acidity, as do alcohol, artificial sweeteners, coffee/tea, drugs/medications, oils (hydrogenated), pepper, and table salt.

The Secret of Longevity

Our greatest desire in life is retaining youth with its grace, beauty, vivacity, and charm. Yet we render ourselves old at forty. Instead of reaching our senior years with a healthy glow, vital energy, and ambition, millions will needlessly die from unnecessary ailments, many before they attain the age of seventy-five. Eighty percent of those who reach sixty-five will be invalids, suffering from catarrhal conditions, rheumatism, arthritis, Bright's disease, diabetes. They will require hearing aids for deafness, glasses for failing vision, dentures for loss of teeth, crutches, canes, and wheelchairs. How does this happen? The answer must be in our lifestyle: eating the refined foods of the conventional American diet, faulty elimination, and never properly cleaning out the body have led us to a state of guaranteed illness.

Ask any young person in their teens or even early twenties if they would like to become eighty or ninety and the answer is more than likely to be a horrified no. We have come to think of old age as a state of decrepitude, not realizing that cleansing and a mucus-free diet hold forth a promise of a longevity that can be joyful every single day.

The real secret of longevity is simply to restrict your food intake to a minimum. From Catholic church records showing that many saints lived to a ripe old age eating only a "handful of food" a day, to modern scientific studies that demonstrate significantly increased longevity in animals on very low-calorie diets, we have clear evidence that limited food intake can extend life.

Thousands of seriously ill people have succeeded in overcoming their ailments through following a non-breakfast plan. Two meals a day has proven ample for the average individual. The breakfast or first meal can be eaten at 10:00 a.m., and the next meal as early as 4:30 p.m. or whatever later time proves more convenient. There are also many followers of a one-meal-a-day plan; they tend to prefer their meal in the late afternoon. With one meal a day, practitioners receive the benefit of a 24-hour fast, since no solid food of any kind is eaten between meals. Water, fruit, and vegetable juices can be taken any time when the main diet consists of starchless vegetables and fruits. With this knowledge you can choose and combine foods correctly.

STUMBLING BLOCKS

In trying to transition to a healthy, life-promoting diet, there are many issues that can cause doubt and confusion. Every day you will be bombarded with contradictory information, and faced with new decisions about how and what to eat. The best you can do in these cases is to let your body tell you what it needs. In addition, you can use the information below to help guide you in your process of transformation.

Coffee, Tea, and Other Stimulants

Many of the beverages and condiments in daily use—such as salt, sugar, spices, alcohol, coffee, tea, cocoa, and tobacco—are quite unhealthy, and many people believe they should be avoided entirely. It is true that these foods stimulate the body more or less at the expense of the vitality and efficiency of the nerves, but they do not produce any mucus, nor do they leave any substantial amount of waste in the body, as do wheat products, starchy foods, and meat, fat, and dairy products. Overall, these beverages and condiments are far less harmful than gluttony, so that compared to overeating they are probably preferable.

Admittedly, alcohol is surely a poison, but the English physician, Dr. S. Graham, certainly struck the nail squarely on the head when he wrote, "A drunkard may become old, but a glutton never."

Cold versus Warm Foods

It is a common belief that the temperature of various foods will affect overall body temperature. Most people will consume hot foods when their skin temperature is cold. They will consume cold foods when their skin temperature is hot. These beliefs are not scientific: food temperatures do not affect the core temperature, which is always constant. A more logical solution to the discomfort we feel from changes in external temperature is to exercise some control over the environment. When our skin temperature is hot we can take a cool shower or use a fan. When our skin temperature is cold we can wear warm clothing or increase our indoor heat to a comfortable level. In both instances, when the skin temperature is maintained at a comfortable level we are free to enjoy the foods to which we are biologically adapted. These foods include mostly raw fruits, with some raw vegetables, nuts, and seeds.

Detox Overload

While it is true that you may experience a more vigorous feeling during the first few days of a fruit diet or other cleansing regimen, feelings of weakness and fatigue can arise quickly, accompanied by headaches and even heart palpitations. These are caused by the loosening and dissolving of poisonous mucus that the body has accumulated over the years through overeating, and which is now being eliminated by the circulation of the bloodstream.

This elimination of poisons can easily cause more systemic disturbances, and unless you are thoroughly convinced of the efficacy of a natural diet, you can become dissuaded at this point, beginning to question, and even lose faith in, this necessary internal purification. These healing crises must be recognized as such, and the healing must carry on. The appearance of a haggard face or a feeling of general depression must not cause you to lose sight of the ultimate goal you are anxious to achieve—good health and longevity.

The amount of mucus and toxic poisons stored up in the deepest tissues of the body is much greater than supposed. Unless we recognize the tremendous importance of a thorough and deep cleansing of the human cesspool, we can very easily become deceived by signs of illness that occur as we are trying to heal. This previously unexplained effect of a very cleansing diet has proven to be a stumbling block for other nutritionists and food experts. They do not realize that without preliminary cleansing—such as the cleanses recommended in this book—the mucus and decomposed protein foods stored in the tissues of the stomach and intestines since early childhood will be dissolved too rapidly by the fresh fruits and simple vegetables. If these toxins are permitted to enter the circulation in their concentrated form, they can cause severe symptoms, and even death. Man's finest natural foods (grapes, apples, peaches, apricots, oranges, grapefruit, bananas, pineapples, figs, dates and a host of others) will be wrongly blamed.

Many people have tried vainly to overcome this stumbling block of toxicity emerging in the midst of a cleansing diet. One student, after living for years on a vegetarian mucus-free diet combined with fasting, ate two pounds of the sweetest vine-ripened grapes and at the same time drank two quarts of freshly pressed grape juice. Almost immediately, he had the sensation that he was dying. Extreme dizziness and heart palpitations ensued, followed by severe pains in the stomach and intestinal region. His vision became affected and he was forced to lie down. After about ten to fifteen minutes, the great event occurred. A mucus-filled foaming diarrhea erupted, together with copious vomiting and acid-smelling mucus, and this was soon followed by the greatest event of all. A feeling of great strength tempted him to perform knee-bending and arm-stretching exercises, which he did without tiring 326 consecutive times. Prehistoric man, living on unfired foods in nature must have had this similar feeling.

Salt

Salt is a relatively new addition to the human diet. Historians have found the earliest evidence of salt mining in Europe and have dated it to about 8,500 years ago. Common salt is an absolute poison; it is an inorganic mineral compound that cannot be assimilated into the human body for nutritional purposes, yet the average American will ingest an unhealthy amount of it annually. Salt is a protoplasmic poison and has been directly linked to human disease symptoms including hypertension, high blood pressure, edema, psychological disorders, gout, and premenstrual syndrome. Humans have no instinctual craving for salt. It is a learned and culturally imposed phenomenon. The consumption of salt is consistent only with the consumption of cooked food. Humans who are consuming the foods to which they are biologically adapted would have no cravings for salt. (This final note on the problems created by the use of salt and should be taken with a grain of salt. Sea salt and Real Salt—salt minerals from the Utah mines—have some profound effects when used in cleansing, but daily consumption should be handled with care.)

THE HEALING FAST

When an animal becomes sick or injured, it instinctively uses nature's divine, curative law of fasting. Yet fasting is the most misunderstood and feared of all the curative agencies. Why is fasting so difficult, so weakening, even dangerous? Volumes have been written on the subject of fasting by self-styled experts, yet few people understand exactly what takes place physiologically and pathologically when the healing spirit—the personal, vital, efficient, unfed body—definitively fasts. The answer is this simple, mathematical, physiological formula:

$$V \text{ (vitality)} = P \text{ (power)} - O \text{ (obstruction)}.$$

Since disease is caused by internal uncleanliness, fasting to get rid of built-up impurities can be very healing. Eating "nourishing" foods during a time of illness is a deleterious practice, causing more harm than good. Disease is merely an effort on the part of nature to start the process of healing by eliminating surplus waste and disease matters from your system. If you would but listen, and heed nature's still voice, you would allow yourself to remain quiet, sleep, and stop eating, so as to give nature a chance to eliminate poisons and repair bodily mechanisms.

Regardless of how miserable, sick, feverish, weak, or desperate you may feel, you will feel better if you stop eating. The instinctive voice of nature speaks to all of her children, both animals and men, teaching them how to experience the highest levels of health, but nature is helpless when you insist on obstructing her good intentions with increased eating, drugs, or painkillers. We soon recognize that humans are the sickest animals on Earth because of their incorrect beliefs in their superior knowledge of food and medicine.

When solid foods of all kinds are discontinued during a fast, the bloodstream, which circulates throughout the entire system every thirty seconds (120 times every hour), starts to dissolve the waste matter and mucus that have been deposited in the tissues. This waste will be found in the stomach and intestinal tract, and especially in any specific organs and tissues that are causing symptoms of illness.

The release of aggregated obstacles in a person's constitution can cause him or her to be overloaded by toxins during an extended fast, which can lead to feelings of weakness and fatigue. This is similar to the experience of a person who switches suddenly from a mainstream diet to a fruit-based diet, as discussed above. It is at this point that a critical stumbling block arises for almost all fasters, because they can become quite ill.

In fact, 80 percent of chronically ill people whose condition has become serious would probably die from a long fast. No faster dies through lack of food, however. They actually suffocate in and from their own wastes. For this reason, you should take the utmost caution. In fact, it would be a crime to recommend a long fast to any unfortunate sick human who is so greatly clogged with "waste" that vitality has practically reached a vanishing point. A special selection of food is probably indicated in this case—not for better nourishment, but for a less aggressive effect in dissolving the mucus and poisons. The right foods will help to slow down the rapid elimination of waste, which could otherwise result in a dangerous situation. Awareness of this fact and proper preparation through living on a well-balanced and carefully selected diet will succeed in making the cleansing fast a pleasure rather than an unpleasant experience.

The length of a fast, the timing between fasts, and even instructions on the proper kinds of food to be eaten between fasts should be individually applied in each case. This is especially true in cases of severe illness or long chronic conditions, where the student's vitality is already depleted and at an extreme low. These precautionary methods must be carefully observed since the quantity of mucus now being dissolved may prove to be greater than the student's vital efficiency.

THE POWER OF CLEANSING

However, if the waste, mucus, and poisons in your already overloaded body are too great and too longstanding, then nature alone cannot help; even fasting indefinitely is hopeless. That is when you need to cleanse the openings of the body. Before proper nutrition can be restored, it is essential that the bloodstream be improved and regenerated so it can successfully carry away the poisons and waste that have been dissolved from the tissues. Cleansing on a regular basis will prevent the buildup of poisons that cause sickness.

Internally we are all identical, with thirty feet of intestines that we never clean, though we brush our teeth once or twice a day at the other end. Just study your own body; there are no secrets. Convince yourself of the absolute truthfulness of cleansing the body on a cellular level and having a mucus-free diet for prevention.

Progress comes through recognition of sickness as a remedial measure. During forty years of experimenting and tests carried out on my own body as well as hundreds of others, all of whom were suffering from so-called incurable conditions (e.g., deafness, partial blindness, and paralysis), I learned that my methods of overcoming disease through cleansing and corrective diet lead to complete results.

Health culture has always been a matter of religion, for the body and spirit are difficult to separate. In the past, the priest and the physician were generally the same person, but these two aspects of our being have been dangerously separated by modern culture. A spiritual blindness has driven present civilization to fancy foods and gluttonous lifestyles, to such an extent that we cannot exist much longer in our present manner. It is becoming rapidly and alarmingly necessary to establish a diet regime according to our bodily requirements. We must close our ears and our minds to the false information fed to us by experts who ignorantly recommend man-made foods that are slowly but surely hastening our end.

SUMMARY

The seemingly healthy person must first pass through a condition of cleansing or sickness, so to speak, or at least an intermediary stage of sickness, before attaining the higher level of health. Properly, man in perfect health should exhale fragrance. The stench of odor, sweat, foul breath, and all body odors are merely indications of the rotting matter that practically all bodies contain.

This is the regulation of human health through our diet, and most importantly, through limiting it. Of course, it is hard to fathom how to function over the long term on such a reduced diet, but let your own experimentation guide you. This is why regular cleansing of the body's nine openings is so important. Your body knows what it needs.

The teachings that follow are old yet new; may they be acceptable to all truth-seekers anxious to participate in the supreme embodiment of abundant, joyous health. The fundamental truth that we must all first learn is the importance of obedience to the laws of nature.

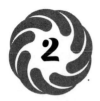

The Nine Openings
of the Body

As Taoists look at the body, it has seven windows, a front door, and a back door—like a temple or a church. The seven windows are the five sense openings in the head: two windows of the eyes, two nostril openings, two ear openings, and one mouth. The front door refers to the genital opening, and the back door to the anus. Together, these comprise the nine openings (fig. 2.1).

The nine openings are the body's thresholds of interaction with the world. Through these orifices flow energy, information, and matter; they allow us to assimilate the outer world into ourselves, and to send aspects of ourselves out into the world. In this chapter, we will explore the physiological functions of each opening, as well as the associated organs and energetic characteristics according to Chinese medicine. Note that the openings have both physical and energetic relationships with their associated organs; when an opening becomes blocked, the body may manifest physical and/or energetic symptoms.

For each of the nine openings, we've included some common ailments that can arise from blockages, and a few different methods of cleansing—including self-massage techniques and physical flushes. Please note, however, that the cleansing information in this chapter is quite general: for specific instructions on how to perform the cleanses and find the appropriate supplements, please see chapter 3.

Each of the nine openings includes certain nearby organs and tissues, which are listed on page 22 in parentheses. In addition, each opening is associated with a specific organ.

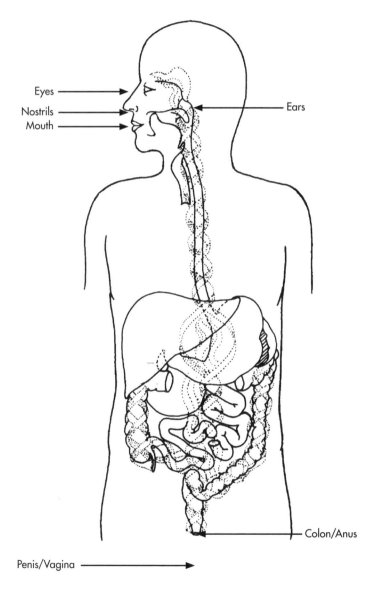

Fig. 2.1. The nine openings of the body

Colon (includes anus, rectum, large intestine) and **lungs**

Genitourinary tract (includes penis, vagina, testicles, ovaries) and **kidneys**

Mouth (includes lips, gums, tongue, throat) and **spleen/ pancreas/heart**

Nostrils (includes nose, sinuses, diaphragm) and **lungs**

Eyes (includes optic nerves, mid-eye, pineal gland, pituitary glands) and **liver**

Ears (includes inner ear, ear drum, adrenal glands) and **kidneys**

THE COLON—THE BACK DOOR

The colon is the most important opening to manage in the physical body (fig. 2.2). Its condition of health or disease has profound effects on a person's overall state of health. Because it is, in part, a sewage system, the colon can quickly become a cesspool when it is neglected or abused. When it is clean and normal we are well and happy; let it stagnate, however, and it will distill the poisons of decay, fermentation, and putrefaction into the blood, poisoning the brain and nervous system so that we become mentally depressed and irritable. It will poison the heart so that we are weak and listless, poison the lungs so that the breath is foul, poison the digestive organs so that we are distressed and bloated, and poison the blood so that the skin is sallow and unhealthy. We will age prematurely, look and feel old, and be overtaken by stiff and painful joints, dull eyes, and a sluggish brain; the pleasure of living will be gone.

Current cultural norms dictate that people should eat three meals a day, but doing so will often overwork and overuse this delicate organ. Since the colon's main function is to digest and process what comes into the body, a constant stream of food precludes a much-needed rest period that would allow for healing to take place. On top of that, the poor quality of some food, and the introduction of chemicals and hormones into the body, put added pressure on the whole

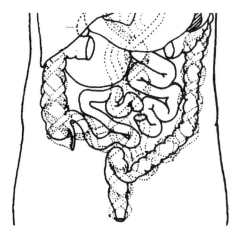

Fig. 2.2. The colon

system. After several decades, these abusive agents wear the colon down, making it vulnerable to cancer or some other health crisis. It is no wonder that colon cancer is one of the most frequently diagnosed cancers in the West.

Characteristics of the Colon

Associated organs: Lungs and skin
Element: Metal
Season/Climate: Autumn (dryness)
Healing sound: Sss-s-s-s-s-s
Parts of the body: Chest, inner arms, thumbs, abdomen
Sense: Smell
Taste: Pungent
Color: White
Negative emotions: Sadness, grief, sorrow
Positive emotions: Righteousness, surrender, courage

Related Organ: Lungs

The colon (yang energy) is energetically connected to the lungs (yin energy). The lungs provide the colon with the energy it needs to defecate and pass unused energy through the anus (fig 2.3).

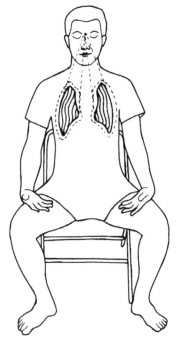

Fig. 2.3. The lungs

The lungs contribute a "distributing-downward" energy to the body's exchange processes. The breath cycle is the most apparent of these exchanges, but the body manages many processes at the same time through other systems. For example, the lungs also govern the circulation of blood and blood vessel health, as well as the body's exchange with its outside environment through the skin.

Common Ailments

Common ailments afflicting the colon include diarrhea, constipation, abdominal pain, and irritable bowel syndrome. Constipation can result when the intestine absorbs too much water and the fecal material is too dry to move easily. Although laxatives may temporarily relieve the symptom of constipation, they do not improve the health of the colon. On the contrary, laxatives poison the muscles of the colon, causing the intestine to twist and twitch like a dying snake.

Diarrhea is the abnormal frequency and liquidity of the feces.

It can be caused by failure of the ileum (the lower part of the small intestine) and the colon to absorb sufficient water. Western medicine has named more than fifty varieties of diarrhea.

Colon-Opening Cleanse

The following therapies will cleanse and detoxify the colon. For details on how to perform these therapies, see chapter 3.

Chi Nei Tsang: Wind Gates, Skin Detox, Scooping technique and Wave technique*

Cellular Cleanse: Bentonite/psyllium drinks, supplements

Flush: Colonics with implants, acidophilus

Additional Cleansing Practices: Dry skin brushing, solar bathing

THE GENITOURINARY TRACT—
THE FRONT DOOR

The genitourinary tract includes the kidneys, the uterus, the bladder, and the urethra, as well as the penis, vagina, ovaries, and testes (see fig. 2.4 on page 26). The urinary system helps to filter and excrete waste and toxins that have been processed by the digestive system. The urinary system—specifically the kidneys—also act as a balancing mechanism, maintaining precise levels of water, pH, and many hormones and minerals that need to be at particular concentrations in the bloodstream. The genital system is responsible for sexual activity as well as the production of sex hormones and reproductive cells.

---

*For more information on Chi Nei Tsang see *Chi Nei Tsang* (Rochester, Vt.: Destiny Books, 2007) and *Advanced Chi Nei Tsang* (Rochester, Vt.: Destiny Books, 2009).

Characteristics of the Genitourinary Tract

Associated organs: Kidneys, bladder, adrenals, genitals, ovaries, testes

Element: Water

Season/climate: Winter (cold)

Healing sound: Choo-oo-oo-oo

Parts of the body: Side of foot, inner leg, chest, groin

Sense: Hearing

Taste: Salty

Color: Black or dark blue

Negative Emotions: Fear, shock

Positive Emotions: Gentleness, stillness, alertness

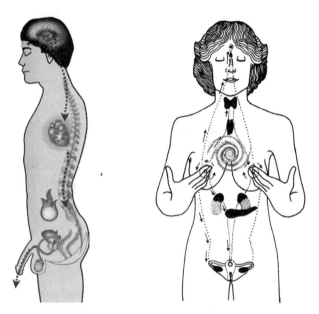

Fig. 2.4. Genital openings and urinary tract

Related Organ: Kidneys

The organ related to the genitourinary tract is, obviously, the kidney. On an energetic level, the kidneys express the base of our spiritual power through the Ming Men point, where the root of chi is stored within the body. The kidneys form the basic yang and yin energies from which all the other organs draw. As the seat of the body's energetic power, the kidneys are an important aspect of the body to keep in balance. Being a water organ yet the source of fire for the whole body, the kidneys must constantly balance themselves between yang and yin energies.

Common Ailments

The urinary tract is vulnerable to irritation and infection; in fact, urinary tract diseases are the second most common kind of infection. The reproductive system may be afflicted by hormone imbalances and infertility, among other ailments. In addition, any imbalances of yin and yang in the organs may have their root in the kidneys, which are the source of all the yin and yang in the body. These imbalances may be expressed in various ways, depending on whether the primary deficiency is one of yin or of yang.

When kidney yin energy is deficient, the body might experience soreness around the kidneys, ringing in the ears, afternoon fevers, or hot, sweaty palms. When kidney yang energy is deficient, the body might experience, again, sore low back and knees, difficulty urinating, decreased energy, decreased sex drive, or an unwillingness to experience any cold feeling. However, because the kidney yin and yang are so intimately connected, disruption of one will ultimately affect the other.

Urinary Tract–Opening Cleanse

The following therapies will cleanse and detoxify the urinary tract. For details on how to perform these therapies, see chapter 3.

Chi Self-Massage: Kidney Tapping, Patting, and
Warming*

---

*For more detailed information on Chi Self-Massage see *Chi Self-Massage* (Rochester, Vt.: Destiny Books, 2006).

Sexual Chi Massage: Genital breathing and compression
Flush: Kidney flush and herbal cleanse

THE MOUTH

The mouth is the next of the openings on our journey (fig. 2.5). Of course, the mouth is a collection of many systems that facilitate our interactions with the outside world. The tongue, teeth, soft and hard palates, and different types of glands all contribute to the function of the mouth. Through the mouth we are able to project our voices, consume food, and vomit if need be. The mouth is the one opening that we make choices about how to fill; it is unlike the other openings in this respect.

Characteristics of the Mouth

Associated Organs: Spleen, pancreas, stomach
Element: Earth
Season/Climate: Indian summer (mild)
Healing Sound: Who-o-o-o-o-o
Parts of the Body: Abdominal area, diaphragm, chest
Sense: Taste
Flavor: Sweet
Color: Yellow

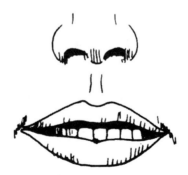

Fig. 2.5. Mouth opening

Negative Emotions: Worry, sympathy, anxiety
Positive Emotions: Fairness, openness, balance

Related Organ: Spleen

The organ related to the mouth is the spleen, which rests behind the stomach in the upper left abdominal region. The spleen's role in traditional Chinese medicine is to help the stomach extract energy from food. This is the process by which the body obtains an important form of chi—Acquired Chi. Acquired Chi supplements our first form of chi, Inborn Chi, which is inherited from our parents.

The spleen chi is a "transporting-upward" energy—like a fountain—that distributes nourishing chi to the rest of the body. The spleen acts as a reservoir for blood and is also a place to break down excess red blood cells. Spleen chi energy also keeps the organs in place, regulates blood flow, and maintains muscle tone. The spleen's health is expressed through the opening of the mouth, and can be assessed by the condition of the lips. Pale, dry lips, for instance, are a sign of poor spleen chi.

The spleen is also viewed as the source of a person's temperament, such that your moods, desires, and inclinations can be very directly expressed through the mouth. That is why the health of this organ is also considered to affect a person's willpower.

Common Ailments

Ailments of the mouth opening may express themselves directly—via mouth sores, gum problems, or salivary duct ailments—or indirectly, via the energy pathways of the spleen. In this case, there may be weakness and fatigue, easy bruising, or low appetite. Poor nutrition and inconsistent meals will adversely affect the health of the spleen, to a point where simply returning to a normal eating pattern may not be enough to fully recover.

Mouth-Opening Cleanse

The following therapies will cleanse and detoxify the mouth. For details on how to perform these therapies, see chapter 3.

Chi Self-Massage: Gums, tongue, teeth

Flush: Olive oil, hydrogen peroxide, baking soda

THE EARS

The ear includes the outer ear and the ear canal, which consists of the eardrum, the hammer, the middle ear, the anvil, the cochlea, and the eustachian tube (fig. 2.6). Collectively, these structures help to filter vibrations and resonations for the hearing system. The ear also acts as an organ of balance for the body, helping us to remain oriented in space.

Characteristics of the Ears

Associated organs: Kidneys, bladder, adrenals

Element: Water

Season/climate: Winter (cold)

Healing sound: Choo-oo-oo-oo

Parts of the body: Side of foot, inner leg, chest, groin

Sense: Hearing

Taste: Salty

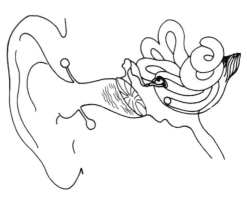

Fig. 2.6. The ear opening

Color: Black or dark blue
Negative Emotions: Fear, shock
Positive Emotions: Gentleness, stillness, alertness

Related Organ: Kidneys

The kidneys govern the two openings of the ears, as well as the opening of the genitourinary tract as described on page 22. Because the kidneys help to filter out waste material from the blood, they can be easily overloaded. If there is more waste in the system than the kidneys can filter, excesses will tend to collect in the kidney ducts and tubules, impairing their function. By flushing the kidneys regularly, we shake out the harmful sediment and help them to operate properly at maximum efficiency.

Common Ailments

Any blockages in the ear canals—such as inflammation, wax build-up, or imbalances between kidney yin and kidney yang—can cause ringing in the ears and loss of hearing. In addition, problems of the inner ear can cause dizziness and vertigo.

The kidneys eliminate toxins after they have been broken down and released from the liver. If the kidneys become overloaded with toxins, they will slow down, resulting in energy loss in the rest of the body. If the kidneys cannot function properly, they may allow too much fluid to be released into the bloodstream, creating high blood pressure.

Ear-Opening Cleanse

The following therapies will cleanse and detoxify the ears. For details on how to perform these therapies, see chapter 3.

Chi Self-Massage: Outer ear, lobes and shells; inner ear, drums
Flush: Ear candling (burning wax candles)

THE NOSTRILS

The nostrils have several vital functions. In addition to allowing us a sense of smell, they protect the lungs in two important ways. When we inhale properly (through the nose and not through the mouth), the nose filters out dirt, preventing it from reaching the lungs. The nose also warms the air, so that very cold air will not injure the lungs, which are quite sensitive.

The nose has three energy meridians running through it: the Large Intestine meridian, the Stomach meridian, and the Governor Channel. Rubbing the nose thus stimulates the stomach and large intestine, strengthens the temperature regulator, and increases hormone secretion. In China, just a few needles inserted on the nose serve as a general anesthetic prior to surgery on any part of the body.

Characteristics of the Nostrils

Associated Organs: Lungs, large intestine, sinuses, skin
Element: Metal
Season/Climate: Autumn (dryness)
Healing Sound: Sss-s-s-s-s-s
Parts of the Body: Chest, inner arms, thumb, diaphragm
Sense: Smell
Taste: Pungent
Color: White
Negative Emotions: Sadness, grief, sorrow
Positive Emotions: Righteousness, surrender, courage

Related Organ: Lungs

The lungs are paired, cone-shaped organs located in the thoracic cavity. They are separated from the heart by the pleural membrane that encloses each lung, and separated from the abdominal cavity by the diaphragm. The lungs mix blood with oxygen and expel used air, including carbon dioxide and other toxins. The diaphragm and inter-costal muscles can control the motion of the lungs.

As previously mentioned, the lungs are the yin metal organ according to the five element system. They have a variety of func-tions, the first of which is to produce lung chi. The lungs govern this chi—along with respiration—down to the cellular level. It is in the cells of the lungs that an individual's internal chi meets up with the chi of the universe, carried in the air. The lungs also control skin and sweat.

Common Ailments

An unhealthy nose will be unable to adequately protect the lungs from frequent colds and infections. In such cases, the sinuses may often be congested, runny, and/or infected. Chronic sinus infections can give rise to many health issues, including headaches, dental problems, and fatigue. A weak nose can also affect the voice, and even the personal-ity. A thin, flat, and unhealthy-looking nose, or a badly shaped nose, can make you less attractive to other people. A strong nose, on the other hand, can help you to have good chi.

The nose is the place where the breath of life enters our bod-ies. Rubbing and massaging the nose will increase the chi and will improve circulation around the nose.

Nostril-Opening Cleanse

The following therapies will cleanse and detoxify the nostrils. For details on how to perform these therapies, see chapter 3.

Chi Self-Massage: Nostrils, bridge, and the sides of the
nose
Flush: Warm salt water

THE EYES

The eyes are the windows of the spirit. In Taoism we regard the eyes as yang energy that guide the chi flow in the whole body. The eyes can greatly affect your personality.

Nowadays people use their eyes much more than in the past to read, watch television, and work with computers, electronics, and microscopes. This strains them a great deal, and drains energy from the eyes as well as from the liver, their associated organ. Since the eyes are connected to the nervous system, they have a special importance, revealing the health of your entire body: through the eyes we can tell which organs are weak and/or toxic (fig. 2.7). Cleansing and massaging the eyes will remove stress from the vital organs.

Some people are born with a lot of white in their eyes—three portions of white to one portion of iris—which can result in a suspicious look. This condition, sometimes called "thief eyes" or "danger attack eyes," can cause people to feel uncomfortable around you. However, this imbalance can often be corrected with the cleanses and exercises described here.*

Characteristics of the Eyes

Associated Organs: Liver and gallbladder
Element: Wood
Season/Climate: Spring (dampness)
Healing Sound: Sh-h-h-h-h-h-h
Parts of the Body: Ribs, inner legs, groin, diaphragm
Sense: Sight
Taste: Sour
Color: Green
Negative Emotions: Anger, aggression
Positive Emotions: Kindness, generosity, forgiveness

---

*For additional information on improving your eyesight and the health of your eyes, see *The Art of Cosmic Vision* (Rochester, Vt.: Destiny Books, 2010), coauthored by Mantak Chia and Robert T. Lewanski.

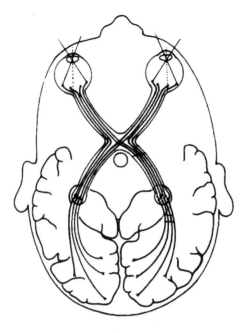

Fig. 2.7. Eye/brain connection

Related Organ: Liver

The liver stores all the toxins, poisons, chemicals, and drugs that the body takes in. Its function is to chemically break down these poisons into less toxic compounds that can be more easily eliminated from the body.

In the practice of Chinese medicine, the liver also stores blood and ensures the smooth flow and direction of chi in the body. As a part of this chi-flowing function, the liver also greatly influences the flow and rhythm of the digestive system. It is also said to contribute to our body's resistance to external pathogenic influences. When the liver is in a state of good health, it is the origin of kindness and resoluteness. It is also believed that the liver influences our ability to plan our lives. Other functions of the liver include controlling the sinews, showing its health on the nails, opening into the eyes, housing the Ethereal Soul (Hun), and affecting dreams.

Common Ailments

When the openings of the eyes become blocked, many vision problems can arise, including macular degeneration, blurry vision, floaters, and near- and far-sightedness. Blockages of the eyes might also be caused by problems in the liver. Because so many toxins are processed by the liver, this organ is frequently overloaded. When the poisonous load becomes too high, the liver's digestive process and other functions are prevented from working properly. The secretion of bile in the gallbladder will likely slow down, leading to the formation of gallstones that can further impair digestive function.

Since the toxins in the liver have built up over a period of time, they must be released slowly, with a well-planned and carefully executed cleansing flush. In addition, the rest of the body should be supported at the same time, with detoxification of the spleen and lymphatic system, and tonification of the kidneys.

Eye-Opening Cleanse

The following therapies will cleanse and detoxify the eyes. For details on how to perform these therapies, see chapter 3.

Chi Nei Tsang: Pumping, Scooping, Patting, and Baking
Chi Self-Massage: Eyeballs, eyelids, sockets, tearing, and sunning
Flush: Epsom salts, olive oil, grapefruit

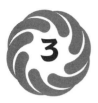

3

Cleanses for
the Nine Openings

This chapter focuses on cleansing the nine openings of the body referred to as the back door (anus), front door (penis and vaginal canal), and the seven windows (two eyes, two ears, two nostrils, and mouth) (fig. 3.1). As a general rule we should keep these areas clean, open, and flowing in order to eliminate any debris or toxins

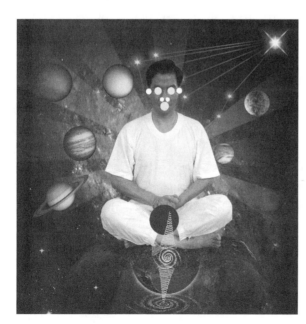

Fig. 3.1. The nine openings are the back door, the front door, and the seven windows.

that have entered or have been stored. During the cleansing process we work to eliminate accumulated toxins and poisons through these nine openings; afterward we consciously seal them to retain their energy.

THE BACK DOOR

The Colon

The key to the health of the back door—and in many ways the health of the whole body—is how well you eliminate the toxins and built-up debris you have ingested. For the colon—which includes the anus, rectum, and the whole lower abdomen—Taoists highly recommend regular cleansing practices to clear out any buildup of toxins. The most important of these practices are colonics and dry skin brushing; also recommended are solar bathing, rectum cleaning, and a natural-sponge face wash. These cleansing practices are described in more detail below.

In general, breathing deeply and mindfully—by expanding the lower abdominals to draw air in and thus expand the lungs, and then flattening the abdominals to push the used air out of the body—helps to activate and repair all of the body's natural eliminative processes. In this way, any type of aerobic exercise will help elimination by activating the lungs, which then activate their paired organ, the colon. Conversely, when you clean out the back door you will also improve your breathing.

If you have never cleaned your colon or rectum out, and have been building up toxins for twenty or thirty or forty years, you can just imagine what have in there. You need to cleanse this area of the body just as you do the other end of the body (the mouth and the teeth). As you cleanse the colon you will start to eliminate a lot of excess body fat and acids.

Colonics

Colonics are a method of flushing the colon with water to clear out impacted food waste and debris. There are two main types of colonics—an open-ended type and a closed-end type. The open-ended colonic involves the insertion into the rectum of a thin-tipped hose, which is connected to a container filled with lukewarm water. Other ingredients, known as *implants*, might be added to the water, including chlorophyll, coffee, garlic, Epsom salts, or a combination of these. A closed-end colonic device is operated by a colon therapist. Its metal insert sends water into the colon and pulls the evacuated debris out.

The process of a colonic is similar to a mouthwash, except that it happens in the colon. You wash the internal skin of the colon and thereby release any blockages. But whereas the closed-end type uses a machine to push water in and flush it back out, the open-ended type relies on gravity and the actual rectal muscles to eliminate the water solution and its accompanying debris. In this book we will be describing methods and practices for open-ended colonics that you can do at home; if you prefer, however, you can have them performed at a professional facility instead (fig. 3.2).

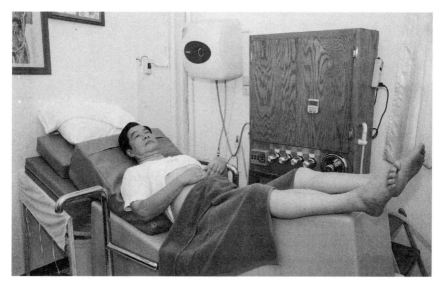

Fig. 3.2. Colonic cleansing at a professional colonic facility

A colonic series consists of one colonic every other day for a week to two weeks. You should do a series every six months to cleanse out your whole body. The only caution is that colonics will draw out from the digestive wall a lot of the natural bacteria that you need to digest food; you will need to include acidophilus supplements so you can culture the bacteria again within the colon.

With an open-ended colonic you will fill up a bucket of water, put it over the toilet to give it gravity, and sit on a special board as you hook tubing up over the toilet (fig. 3.3).* As you slowly release water from the tip of the bucket tubing into the rectum, you can massage your abdomen and also do light aerobic exercises to help your body eliminate (fig. 3.4).

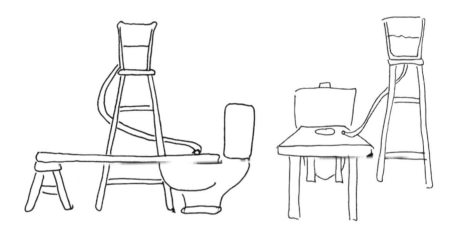

Fig. 3.3. Set-up for an open-ended colonic
that can be self-administered

One of the problems with the colon is that human beings stand upright—unlike other animals, who are on all fours. Because of our upright stance, our bodies have to move waste *up* the body in the ascending colon, against gravity. This means that someone with deficient chi may become constipated, further exacerbating the person's

*Please see the resources section on pages 149–51 for details on where to purchase a colonic board, often called a *colema* board.

unhealthy condition. Once you are cleaning your colon regularly you start to realize that how you defecate is important. Odors, gas, and even the way you sit become important details of your daily life. If you have a very cleansing diet that includes a lot of chlorophyll, for instance, there will be no smell at all to defecation, or any gas either. Much of the gas and the smells we associate with our bowels come actually from improper foods that do not agree with the body. It is the horrible combinations of what we put into our bodies—the animal products, the acidic products, the sugars, and starches—that create a chemical reaction as they start to break down; this leads to explosions of gas.

The best position for defecating is a squatting posture. In much of Asia, they do not have toilet seats because they squat on their haunches instead. This is a much more hygienic method because you do not physically sit on anything, so there is no risk of germ transmission. Many traditional Asian cultures also use water to wash the anus instead of toilet paper, which has a tendency to get matted up in the buttocks and prevent proper drying.

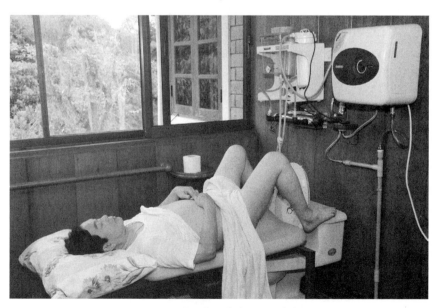

Fig. 3.4. Massaging the abdomen while using a
self-operating colonic board

Colonic Cleansing

1. Set colonic board* hood on toilet and board on stool or use a professional colonic specialist.
2. Hook up tubing to bucket; then fill it with warm water and rinse. Check water release.
3. Insert rectal tip into tube in board hood. Place pad on board and lie on your back on the board with your buttocks on the hood.
4. Apply rectal gel and insert rectal tip into anus.
5. Relax. Release tube clamp. Allow water to flow freely.
6. Massage the left side of your lower abdomen—the descending colon—in an upward direction (against its normal direction of flow) toward the bottom of the rib cage. Work through any tender spots. Continue across the transverse colon just below the rib cage, and then down the right side, which is the ascending colon.
7. When it becomes necessary to evacuate, relieve the bowels by expelling water. Feces will normally bypass the tip without pushing it out.
8. Repeat steps 5–7 a few times until the bucket is empty (about 45 minutes). Do not flush the toilet during the entire colonic. Instead, look at what comes out (it will be black/green feces).
9. To finish, clamp the tube, remove the tip, and slip out from the board. Wash the board; then sit on the toilet to defecate.
10. Clean yourself; then collect energy at your navel point as follows. Starting at the navel, men should spiral the energy outward in a clockwise direction, making 36 revolutions. Once you have completed the clockwise revolutions, spiral inward in a counterclockwise direction 24 times, ending and collecting the energy at the navel.

    Women should make the same action, but begin by spiraling the energy out from the navel in a counterclockwise direction and spiraling back to the navel in a clockwise direction.

---

*See the resources section at the end of the book for sources of colonic boards, tubing, and other necessary colonic supplies.

Do two colonics per day for seven days, or one colonic every other day for two weeks.

Implants

Implants are additives that are placed in the water during a colonic. They can be used to nourish the body and/or aid cleansing. They can be combined or taken individually.

- Chlorophyll liquid concentrate (½ cup of liquid squeezed from green grass)
- Coffee (2 tablespoons ground coffee simmered in 1 quart of water for 15 minutes. Strain and add to bucket.)
- Garlic (3 cloves blended and strained into bucket)
- Lemon juice (¼ cup strained into bucket)
- Saline (1 tablespoon of sun-dried sea salt dissolved into bucket)
- Epsom salts (1 tablespoon dissolved into bucket)
- Glycothymoline (8 ounces per 5 gallons of water)
- Acidophilus (1 quarter of bottle into bucket)

After your colonic series ends, eat only whole fruits and vegetables for two days. They can be steamed or cooked into soup. Also take acidophilus twice a day for two weeks.

Dry Skin Brushing

In Chinese medicine, the skin is often called a "third lung" because of its connection to the lungs and large intestine. For this reason, a colon cleanse also includes opening and cleaning out the pores of the skin with dry skin brushing and solar bathing. Skin brushing should be done on a regular basis for maintenance, youthfulness, and longevity, and should be included in the periodic colon cleanse (see fig. 3.5 on page 44).

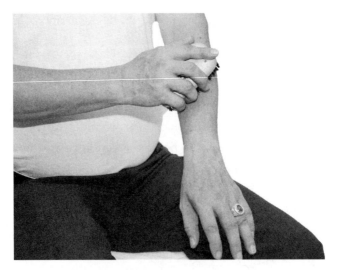

Fig. 3.5. Dry skin brushing

Use a bristle brush or loofah brush before your morning bath and before bed at night. Gently brush with strokes from outer points of the body to the center. The skin should glow with a pink color; it should not turn red. The total process takes about 3 minutes.

1. Do the Inner Smile meditation (see appendix 2 for directions on how to do the Inner Smile meditation).
2. Beginning at the sole of the right foot, brush from sole of foot up the entire leg to the groin. Use short, quick strokes or long sweeping strokes toward the heart. Use as many strokes as are needed to brush the front, back, and sides of the leg.
3. Repeat step 2 on the left leg.
4. Brush buttocks, hips, lower back, and abdomen with circular motions.
5. Brush the left arm from the hand up to the shoulder, then circle the left breast. Make sure to brush the top, bottom, and sides of the arm.
6. Repeat step 5 on the right arm and breast.
7. Brush across the upper back, then down the front, back, and sides of the torso. Cover entire skin surface once.

8. Use a softer brush on the face. Begin in the center of the face and stroke outward. Brush down the sides of the face and neck.
9. To finish, jump into the shower and feel a light, tingling sensation over your body.
10. Clean and dry your body, then collect energy at the navel point as follows. Starting at the navel, men should spiral the energy outward in a clockwise direction, making 36 revolutions. Once you have completed the clockwise revolutions, spiral inward in a counterclockwise direction 24 times, ending and collecting the energy at the navel.

    Women should make the same action, but begin by spiraling the energy out from the navel in a counterclockwise direction and spiraling back to the navel in a clockwise direction.

Solar Bathing

Expose your entire body to the open air to absorb vitamin D.

1. Use the Inner Smile meditation to smile down to your organs (see appendix 2 for directions).
2. Lie down naked in a secluded area, absorbing fresh air and the sun's rays for 10 minutes on each side (fig. 3.6).

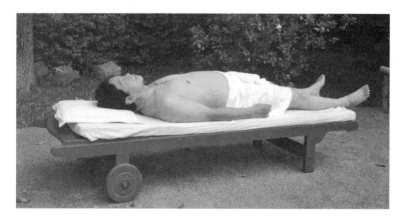

Fig. 3.6. Solar bathing

3. Work up to 30 minutes on each side by adding 5 minutes each day.

4. Collect energy at the navel. Do the Six Healing Sounds. (See appendix 3 for directions on how to practice the Six Healing Sounds.)

Rectum Cleansing

After defecating on the toilet, it's a good time to clean the rectum. Men can also massage the prostate at this time.

You will need the following supplies: a surgical glove or plastic finger cot, castor oil, Dr. Bronner's pure castile soap.

1. While sitting on the toilet after completing your bowel movement, cover your middle finger with a finger cot or surgical glove and insert it into your rectum. Clean out your rectum, massaging the upper roof of the rectum wall. This massage will effectively massage the prostate, if you have one.

2. Remove your finger, keeping the finger cot on, and apply castor oil. Re-insert the finger into your rectum and clean again. It may take several rounds of cleaning to complete the process, as you are likely to experience a few more bowel movements while you do it.

3. Remove the glove and clean your hands with pure castile soap.

Natural Sponge Face Wash

You can perform this facial wash any time your skin feels tight or dry. When done on a regular basis it can prevent dry skin and signs of aging. You will need a natural sea sponge and cool purified water for this practice.

1. Soak the sea sponge in purified water and gently apply it to your face. You can gently clean, rub, and massage your skin (fig. 3.7).

2. After completing the wash do not dry your face. Instead, allow it

to dry naturally, so that your facial skin will absorb the purified water.

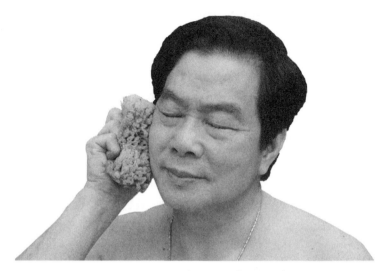

Fig. 3.7. Natural sponge face wash

Celluar Cleansing

While you are doing a colonic cleanse, we suggest you do a cellular cleanse at the same time to improve your results. This cleanse consists of a 7–14-day fast, during which you ingest only vegetable broths and specific herbs and supplements. These supplements will activate the energy and debris in your system, so that they are more easily removed by the colonics.

This cellular cleanse came from natural health pioneer Victor Irons over ninety years ago; it recommends oral bentonite and psyllium for cleansing the colon, and taking supplements to strengthen and build up the cells. Together, the supplements—including chlorophyll, digestive enzymes, and essential fatty acids—draw toxins out of individual cells and into the intestinal system, where they can be effectively eliminated. Then psyllium and bentonite help to pull the debris off of the colon walls, which allows you to eliminate this caked up material from the body.

Bentonite is a form of clay that was once blown into the sky by volcanic action, then sifted down to earth, where it collected in layers or veins that can be mined. Its action is due to three things. First, its large and varied mineral content gives it a negative electrical charge, which attracts positively charged particles. In the human body, much of the toxic poisons are positively charged. Second, the minuteness of the particles of bentonite give it a very large surface area in proportion to its volume, thus enabling it to pick up many times its own weight in positively charged particles such as body acid debris. Third, to obtain maximum effectiveness in the human body, it should be in a liquid colloidal gel state. For information on where to buy colloidal bentonite and the other supplements recommended in this cleanse, see the resources section beginning on page 146.

Clays have been used as natural medicines for thousands of years. Nutrition pioneer Weston A. Price found it in common use among the Yucatan Indians of Mexico, for instance. When an Indian had a cut, bruise, abrasion, or irritation, he would immediately make a "mudpie" with a certain clay and apply it to the affected area to help it heal. The Yucatan people also took clay internally; when they did not feel "up to par" generally, they would immediately go to this special clay and mix it into a solution with water and drink it. This seemed to relieve whatever symptoms were present, and in a great many cases, these people seemed to live to a ripe old age.

Indigenous people from places as diverse as the Andes, Central Africa, and Australia have also been known to ingest clay. In many cases people regularly dipped their food into clay to prevent a "sick stomach."

The Cellular Cleanse (with Colonics)

This is a liquid fasting cell cleanse that uses bentonite, psyllium, and various supplements for a period of 7–14 days, with a colonic every other day for greatest results. You should eat nothing for the 7–14 days of the cleanse, but you may drink herbal teas or vegetable broths.

Note that you should always consult your physician about your ability to complete this cleanse. If you are able, we recommend that you do this cleanse 2–4 times a year.

You will need the following supplies for this cleanse: a pint jar, apple juice, apple cider vinegar, honey, bentonite, psyllium seed husks, and the supplements listed in the table on page 50. Sources for purchasing these supplements are listed in the resources section. You will also need the colonic supplies listed in the resources section.

The cleanse consists of two drinks mixed separately. Drink them in succession 5 times per day.

1st Drink

Place all of the ingredients in jar. Shake for 15 seconds. Drink quickly.

> 2 ounces apple juice, lemon juice, or lime juice for flavor
>
> 8 ounces pure water
>
> 1 tablespoon colloidal bentonite
>
> 1 teaspoon psyllium

2nd Drink

Place all ingredients in pint jar. Shake, and drink quickly.

> 10 ounces pure water
>
> 1 tablespoon apple cider vinegar or other vinegar
>
> 1 teaspoon honey or pure maple syrup

Supplements

Along with the two cleansing drinks you will need to take the supplements listed in the following table 4 times a day on the days specified. You should separate the cleansing drinks and the supplements by 1.5 hours. For example, if you take the cleansing drinks at 7:00 a.m., you should take the supplements at 8:30.

SUPPLEMENT SCHEDULE (4 times per day)

	Day 1	Day 2	Days 3, 7, & 14
Chlorophyll gel tablets	12	18	24
Vitamin C tablets	200 mg	200 mg	800 mg
Pancreatin tablets	6	6	6
Beet tablets	2	2	2
Dulse tablets	1	1	1
Enzymatic tablets	2	2	2
Niacin tablets	50 mg	100 mg	200 mg
Wheat germ oil tablets	1	1	1

THE FRONT DOOR

The Urinary Tract and Genitals

For the urinary tract, which includes the penis, prostate, vagina, testicles, ovaries, bladder, and kidneys, most of the cleansing practices focus on the kidneys. Because they are the source of all the yin and yang in the body, the repository of Ancestral Chi, and the source of sexual energy, the kidneys are a vital energy center that needs to be kept in good health. To help to keep the kidneys clean and in prime condition, Taoists highly recommend herbal teas, vaginal douches, vegetable cleanses, and Sexual Chi Massage on a regular basis. These will help to clear out any debris, blockages, and built-up toxins from the urinary tract.

Cleansing the Kidneys

The kidneys are extremely delicate, blood-filtering organs that congest easily. Dehydration, poor diet, weak digestion, stress, and an irregular lifestyle can all contribute to the formation of kidney stones. Most kidney grease/crystals/stones, however, are too small to be detected through modern diagnostic technology, including ultrasounds or X-rays. They are often called "silent" stones and do not seem to bother people much. When they grow larger, though, they can cause considerable distress and damage to the kidneys and the rest of the body.

To prevent kidney problems and kidney-related diseases, it is best to eliminate kidney stones before they can cause a crisis. You can easily detect the presence of sand or stones in the kidneys by pulling the skin under your eyes sideways toward the cheekbones. Any irregular bumps, protrusions, red or white pimples, or discoloration of the skin indicates the presence of kidney sand or kidney stones.

Herbal Kidney Cleanse

The following herbs, when taken daily for a period of twenty to thirty days, can help to dissolve and eliminate all types of kidney stones, including uric acid, oxalic acid, phosphate, and amino acid stones. If you have a history of kidney stones, you may need to repeat this cleanse a few times, at intervals of six weeks.

Marjoram (1 ounce)
Cat's claw (1 ounce)
Comfrey root (1 ounce)
Fennel seed (2 ounces)
Chicory herb (2 ounces)
Uva ursi (2 ounces)
Hydrangea root (2 ounces)
Gravel root (2 ounces)
Marshmallow root (2 ounces)
Goldenrod herb (2 ounces)

❂ *Directions*

1. Thoroughly mix all the herbs together and put them in an airtight container. You may put them in the refrigerator.
2. Before bedtime, put 3 tablespoons of the herb mixture in 2 cups of water. Cover, and let it sit overnight.
3. The following morning, bring the concoction to a boil, then strain it. (If you forget to soak the herbs in the evening, boil the mixture in the morning and let it simmer for 5 to 10 minutes before straining.)
4. Drink a few sips at a time in 6 to 8 portions throughout the day. This tea does not need to be taken warm or hot, but do not refrigerate it. Also, do not add sugar or sweeteners. Leave at least one hour after eating before taking your next sips.
5. Repeat this procedure for twenty days.

If you experience discomfort or stiffness in the area of the lower back, this is because mineral crystals from kidney stones are passing through the ducts of the urinary system. Normally, the release is gradual and does not significantly change the color or texture of the urine, but any strong smell or darkening of the urine that occurs during the kidney cleanse indicates a major release of toxins from the kidneys.

Important: Support your kidneys during this cleanse by drinking extra amounts of water, a minimum of six to eight glasses per day. However, if the urine is a dark yellow color, you will need to drink more than that amount.

❂ Bone Marrow Soup Kidney Cleanse

Make a bone marrow soup with the following ingredients, and drink it on a regular basis to maintain kidney performance and health.

Cracked organic beef bone (knuckles), marrow exposed

Seaweed (hijiki or nori)
Garlic
Added Vegetables: Carrots, onions, zucchini, celery,
    burdock root, daikon radish

Kidney Tonics

The following preparations tonify the kidneys and increase their ability to filter impurities from the blood.

- Cranberry juice (unsweetened) with an equal amount of purified water
- 1 to 2 lemons juiced in purified water

Male Sexual Chi Massage

Internal Belly Breath

1. Place middle fingers 1.5" below navel.
2. Inhale into fingertips.
3. Exhale and release.
   Repeat 81 times.

Kidney Warmer

1. Stand with both feet firmly on the floor and rub hands together briskly until they are warm.
2. Place hands on the low back over the kidneys and bend forward slightly.
3. Inhale, pulling energy up from the left and right sides of the anus into the left and right kidneys, testicles, and other organs.
4. Exhale, and allow the kidneys to deflate.
5. Repeat steps 1, 2, & 3.
   Repeat 36 times.

⊙ Male Power Lock

Inhale into the crown of the head 3 times.

⊙ Silk Cloth Massage

1. With a silk cloth, massage your genitals, perineum, and sacrum.
2. Starting at the navel, spiral the energy outward in a clockwise direction, making 36 revolutions. Once you have completed these revolutions, spiral inward in a counterclockwise direction 24 times, ending and collecting the energy at the navel.
3. Feel the testicles loose and full of chi.

⊙ Testicle Finger Massage

1. Hold testicles in both hands.
2. Press thumbs on testicles.
3. Massage them 36 times in a clockwise direction, then 36 times counterclockwise.
4. Roll them left, right, back and up, 36 times.

⊙ Testicle Palm Massage

1. Hold testicles in the palm of your left hand.
2. Lightly press your palm against your testicles, and rub gently in a clockwise direction 36 times.
3. Then rub in a counterclockwise direction 36 times.
4. Warm hands by rubbing them briskly together, then hold testicles in right hand.
5. Repeat steps 2 and 3 with the right hand.
6. Draw energy up to the crown of your head.

❂ *Elongating the Ducts*

1. Cup testicles in your hands. Use the thumb and forefinger of each hand to trace the seminal ducts up and down.
2. Draw energy to the crown of your head.

❂ *Duct-Stretching Massage*

1. Grasp the seminal ducts between your thumbs and forefingers.
2. Gently pull testicles out, stretching the ducts (fig. 3.8).
3. Massage Testicles.
    Repeat 36 times and draw energy up.

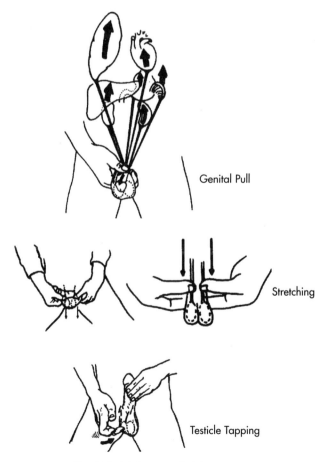

Genital Pull

Stretching

Testicle Tapping

Fig. 3.8. Male sexual chi massage

☯ *Genital Pull*

1. Encircle the base of the penis with your thumb and index finger.
2. Pull entire groin downward in a clockwise circular motion while you focus on pulling your internal organs upward.
3. Hold, then release drawing energy up to crown.

Repeat 36 times clockwise, then counterclockwise.

☯ *Penis Massage*

1. Hold the base of your penis between the thumbs and forefingers of both hands.
2. Draw energy up.
3. Massage penis along the left side, right side, and midline from the base to the tip 36 times.

☯ *Testicle Tapping*

1. Inhale and pull your energy up.
2. Hold your breath, clench your teeth, contract your perineum and anus.
3. Lift penis with your left hand and lightly tap your right testicle with your right hand 9 times.
4. Exhale and rest, drawing energy up your spine.
   Repeat steps 3 and 4, switching hands and this time tapping your left testicle.

☯ Female Sexual Chi Massage

☯ *Belly Breath*

1. Place middle fingers 1.5" below navel and inhale into fingertips.
2. Exhale and release.
   Repeat 81 times.

⊙ *Kidney Warmer*

1. Rub hands together briskly until they're warm, and place your palms on your back over the kidneys. Bend body forward slightly.
2. Inhale. Pull up on the left and right sides of your anus, drawing energy into your left and right to kidneys.
3. Exhale. Deflate kidneys. Rub hands together briskly and when they're warm, place them on the kidneys.
   Repeat 36 times.

⊙ *Female Power Lock*

Inhale into the crown of the head 3 times.

⊙ *Silk-Cloth Massage*

1. Through a silk cloth, press 3 fingers onto the outside of the vagina to massage the perineum, vaginal muscles, and sacrum.
2. Starting at the navel, spiral the energy outward in a counterclockwise direction, making 36 revolutions.
3. Spiral inward in a clockwise direction 24 times, ending and collecting the energy at the navel.
4. Feel enlarged breasts and moist vagina.

⊙ *Breast Massage*

1. Sit on the floor, naked and cross-legged so that you feel a firm pressure against your vagina. Pull up your anus, drawing chi up along the spine.
2. Pull up the left and right sides of the anus and bring chi up to your nipples.
3. Place your tongue against your palate, and warm your hands by rubbing them together briskly.

4. Place your palms on your breasts so that the second joint of each middle finger is on the nipple. Rub in gentle circles 36 times clockwise, then 36 times counterclockwise.

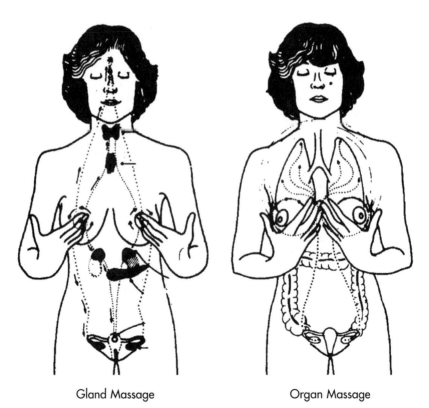 Gland Massage

1. Beginning with your middle fingers on the nipples, trace spiraling circles outward until you surround the whole breast (fig. 3.9). Then spiral back in toward the nipples.
2. Draw chi from your energized clitoris up to your head, activating your pineal and pituitary glands.
3. Continue massaging, and activate the thyroid and parathyroid glands. Draw the chi from these four glands down into the thymus to activate it.

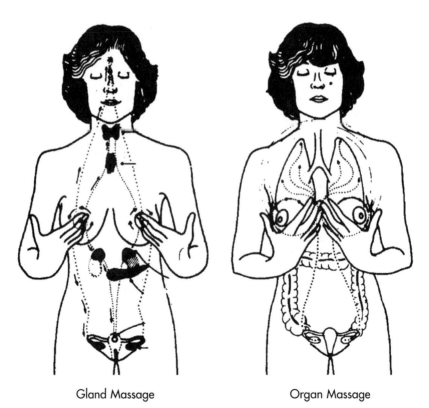

Gland Massage   Organ Massage

Fig. 3.9. Female sexual chi massage

4. Allow all of this glandular chi to accumulate and draw it into your breasts, then down to the pancreas.
5. From the pancreas, let the accumulated chi flow back to the breasts.
6. Activate the adrenal glands and bring their energy into the breasts.

🌀 Organ Massage

1. Warm hands by rubbing them together, and cover your breasts. Massage them in gentle circles.
2. Feel chi from the thymus activating the lungs. Draw accumulating lung chi into the breasts.
3. Continue massaging, and activate your heart. Draw its chi into your breasts.
4. Repeat with spleen, kidneys, and liver, drawing all the accumulating energy into the breasts.
4. Cover your vagina with one hand, and allow the chi in the breasts to expand into the nipples.
5. With concentration, let the accumulated breast energy drop into the ovaries. Feel pulsation of vagina, as if it is opening and closing.
6. Draw chi into the Ovarian Palace—a point in the cervix, about 3 inches below the navel. Gently squeeze to tense the cervix and hold the energy there.
7. Relax and absorb the accumulated chi.

🌀 Ovaries Massage

1. Warm the hands and place them on a silk cloth over the ovaries. Massage 36 times in both directions, stimulating the breasts and clitoris.*

---

*You can continue this exercise with vaginal egg exercises, which strengthen the muscles of the vagina. For complete directions for the vaginal egg exercise, see *Healing Love through the Tao* (Rochester, Vt.: Destiny Books, 2005).

THE SEVEN WINDOWS

The following pages include cleansing programs and exercises for each of the seven windows. Most of the exercises can be performed daily for maintenance, while the more intense cleansing programs may be recommended only once or twice per year.

The Eyes

Because the eyes are governed by the liver, therapies for cleansing the eyes are largely focused on that organ and its yang counterpart, the gallbladder. Good practices include regular chi self-massage eye exercises and eyewashes, as well as periodic liver and gallbladder flushes, herbal teas, and vegetable cleanses. These will help to clear out any debris or blockages, and any buildup of toxins in the eye system.

Liver and Blood Purifier Tea

The herbs listed below are best taken as a tea for 10 days during each change of season, and at times of acute illness. These are the most prominent herbs for improving liver function and maintaining clean blood. For maximum effectiveness, use all of these herbs together.*

> Dandelion root (1 ounce)
> Comfrey root (½ ounce)
> Licorice root (1 ounce)
> Agrimony (1 ounce)
> Wild yam root (1 ounce)
> Barberry bark (1 ounce)
> Bearsfoot (1 ounce)
> Tanners oak bark (1 ounce)
> Milk thistle herb (1 ounce)

---

*This recipe is from Andreas Moritz, *The Liver and Gallbladder Miracle Cleanse* (Berkeley, Calif.: Ulysses Press, 2007).

1. Mix the dry herbs together and add 2 tablespoons of the mixture to 24 ounces of water.
2. Let it sit for 6 hours or overnight.
3. Bring the mixture to a boil, letting it simmer for 5 to 10 minutes before straining. (If you forget to prepare this tea the night before, bring the mixture to a boil in the morning, let it simmer as indicated above, and strain it.)
4. Drink 2 cups per day on an empty stomach.

 ## Steamed Salad Liver Cleanse

To cleanse the liver, eat nothing but the vegetables listed below for 2–3 days. The vegetables should be lightly steamed.

Beets and beet greens
Sprouts
Kale
Romaine lettuce
Celery

 ## Liver and Gallbladder Flush

After cleaning your kidneys, lungs, spleen, pancreas, and intestines, you need to cleanse your liver, gallbladder, and bile ducts from gallstones and your large intestine from all residues to flush out all dead parasites and improve your overall health. You can expect your allergies to disappear, too. It eliminates shoulder, neck, upper arm, and upper back pain. You will have more energy and well-being.*

You will need the following ingredients listed on page 62:

---

*This recipe is from Hulda Clark, Ph.D., N.D., *The Cure For All Cancers* (San Diego, Calif.: ProMotion Publishing, 1995).

6 quarts of apple juice

4 tablespoons Epsom salts

$^1/_2$ cup cold-pressed olive oil

$^2/_3$ to $^3/_4$ cup freshly squeezed pink grapefruit juice

4 to 8 500-mg Ornithine capsules

You will also need a large plastic straw, a pint jar with a lid, and a 24-ounce bottle or jar.

⚙ Preparation

For 6 days prior to your flush, drink 32 ounces of apple juice per day; you can dilute it with any amount of water. Malic acid in the apple juice will soften gallstones and make their passage through the bile ducts easier. If the juice causes diarrhea, it will be a result of stagnant bile being released by the liver and gallbladder. Drink the apple juice slowly throughout the day, two hours after meals, and not in the evening. Use organic apple juice, concentrate, or apple cider.

Choose a day like Saturday for the cleanse so that you will be able to rest the next day. Take no medicines, vitamins, or pills that you can do without; they could prevent success. Stop any other herbs the day before. Eat a non-fat breakfast and lunch such as cooked cereal with fruit, fruit juice, bread and preserves or honey (no butter or milk), baked potato or other vegetables with salt only. This allows the bile to build up and develop pressure in the liver, which will push out more stones.

⚙ The Flush

1. Do not eat or drink after 2:00 p.m. If you break this rule you could feel quite ill later. Get your Epsom salts ready. Mix 4 tablespoons of Epsom salts in the 24-ounce jar with 3 cups water. This makes 4 servings, ¾ cup each. Put the jar in the refrigerator.

2. At 6:00 p.m. drink 1 serving (¾ cup) of the Epsom salts. If you did

not prepare this ahead of time, mix 1 tablespoon in ¾ cup water now. You may add ½ teaspoon vitamin C powder to improve the taste. You may also drink a few mouthfuls of water afterward or rinse your mouth. Get the olive oil and grapefruit out to warm up.

3. At 8:00 p.m. repeat by drinking another ¾ cup of the Epsom salts. You have not eaten since 2:00, but you will not feel hungry. The timing is critical for success; do not be 10 minutes early or late.

4. At 9:45 p.m. pour ½ cup (measured) olive oil into the pint jar. Squeeze the grapefruit by hand into the measuring cup. Remove pulp with fork. You should have at least ½ cup of juice, though up to ¾ cup is best. Add this to the olive oil. Close the jar tightly with the lid and shake hard until watery (only fresh grapefruit does this).

5. At 10:00 p.m. drink the potion you have mixed. Take 4 ornithine capsules with the first sips to make sure you will sleep through the night. Take 8 if you already suffer from insomnia. Drinking through a large plastic straw helps it go down easier. Take it to your bedside, but drink it standing up. Get it down within 5 minutes.

6. Lie down immediately. You might fail to get stones out if you do not. The sooner you lie down the more stones you will get out. As soon as the drink is down walk to your bed and lie down flat on your back with your head up high on the pillow. Try to think about what is happening in the liver. Try to keep perfectly still for at least 20 minutes. You may feel a train of stones traveling along the bile ducts. There is no pain because the bile duct valves have been relaxed by the Epsom salts. Go to sleep, as you may fail to get stones out if you do not.

7. The next morning at 6:00 a.m. (not before) take your third dose of Epsom salts. If you have indigestion or nausea wait until it is gone before drinking the Epsom salts. Go back to bed.

8. At 8:00 a.m. take your fourth dose of Epsom salts. You may go back to bed, though you can expect to have one or more bowel movements with diarrhea.
9. At 10:00 a.m., after 2 more hours, you may eat. Start with fruit juice. Half an hour later eat fruit. One hour later you may eat regular food but keep it light. By supper you should feel recovered.

Expect diarrhea in the morning. Use a flashlight to look for gallstones in the toilet with the bowel movement. Look for the green kind since this is proof they are genuine gallstones, not food residue. Only bile from the liver is pea green. The bowel movement sinks but the gallstones float because of the cholesterol inside. Roughly count the tan and green ones; you will need to total 2,000 stones before the liver is clean enough to permanently rid you of allergies or upper back pains. The first cleanse may rid you of them for a few days, but as the stones from the rear travel forward, they give you the same symptoms again. You may repeat this cleanse at 2 weeks intervals, but never cleanse when you are ill.

Eye Wash

For this eye wash you will need an eye wash cup, purified water, and fresh squeezed lemon juice or hydrogen peroxide.

1. Fill the eye wash cup with purified water and 2–3 drops of fresh squeezed lemon juice or hydrogen peroxide.
2. Wash each eye 2–3 times (fig. 3.10).
3. You can repeat this wash any time your eyes feel tight, red, or dry.

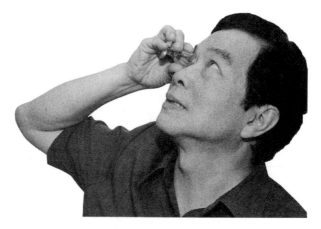

Fig. 3.10. Eye wash

 Chi Self-Massage Eye Exercises

 Eyeball Massage

1. Close your eyes. Use your fingertips to gently massage your eyeballs through your closed eyelids, making clockwise circles 6 to 9
times.
2. Repeat the massage, this time making counterclockwise circles 6
to 9 times (fig. 3.11).
3. Gently massage the area around the eyelids 6 to 9 times.

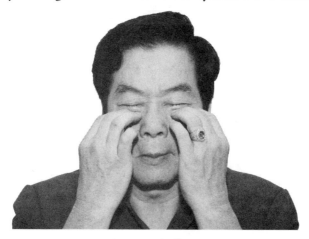

Fig. 3.11. Eyeball massage

✪ *Eyelid Pulling*

Use your thumb and index finger to gently pinch your eyelids. Pull them up and release them 6 to 9 times (fig. 3.12).

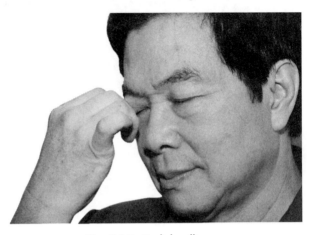

Fig. 3.12. Eyelid pulling

✪ *Eye-Socket Massage*

Bend your index fingers and thumbs, and use the knuckles to rub the upper and lower bones of the eye sockets 6 to 9 times (fig. 3.13).

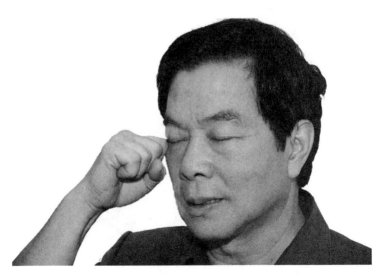

Fig. 3.13. Eye-socket massage

✺ *Eye Tearing*

1. Hold your index finger up about eight inches in front of your eyes, or put a dot on the wall five or six feet away from you (fig. 3.14).

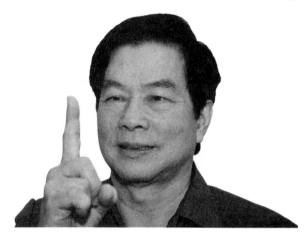

Fig. 3.14. Eye tearing

2. Stare intently at the dot or finger without blinking, until you feel like a fire is burning in your eyes and they begin to tear. The Taoists believe these tears will burn toxins out of your body.
3. Rub your hands briskly together until they are warm; close your eyes and cover your eye sockets with your palms. Feel the hand chi absorbing into your eyes (fig. 3.15).

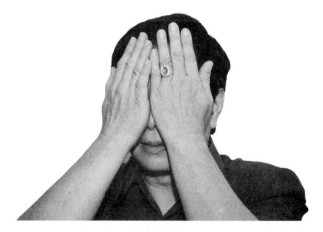

Fig. 3.15. Eyeball cupping

⊙ *Eyeball Pulling and Pressing*

Pulling and pressing the eyeballs will exercise the organs, senses, glands, and the brain. This is also the best exercise for the eye muscles, which can become weak when we don't exercise them, contributing to poor eyesight.

1. With the eyes still closed and cupped by the palms from the eye tearing exercise above, inhale. Contract your anus and sexual organs, and try to pull your eyeballs backward into their sockets.
2. Contract middle of your anus and the middles of your eyeballs.
3. Contract the front of the anus and the tops of the eyeballs.
4. Contract the back of the anus and the bottoms of the eyeballs.
5. Contract right side of the anus and right sides of the eyeballs.
6. Contract the left side of the anus and the left sides of the eyeballs.

This exercise strengthens not only the eyes, but also the pituitary and pineal glands, and the inner ear including the eardrum and ear canal. When you pull the eyeballs in and upward and look toward the crown, you are exercising the upper muscles and stimulating the pituitary and pineal glands. When you contract and pull in the middle of your eyeballs, you are exercising the back of the eye muscles and the inner ear. When pulling in the outer corners of the eyes, you are strengthening the side eye muscles and the ear canals and the eardrums. When pulling in the inner corners of the eyes, you are strengthening the inner side muscles, the tear ducts, and the nose. When pulling in the lower parts of the eyes, you are pressing the lower part of the ear canals and the nervous system.

THE EARS

For the ears, which are our windows to the vibrational universe, the Taoists recommend regular practice of several exercises. These exercises will help to clear any debris or blockages from the outer ear, inner ear, eardrum, adrenal glands, and kidneys.

 ## Ear Candling

For this cleanse, you will need a partner, two ear candles, a bowl of water, scissors, matches, toothpicks, and a disposable aluminum pie tin.

1. Place your partner in a comfortable side-lying position.
2. Cut a dime-size hole in the pie tin. The pie tin will serve to catch any wax, should some drip from the outside of the candle.
3. Insert the candle through the hole in the pie tin (fig. 3.16). Light the large end of the candle, and set the small end firmly in your partner's ear canal. The candle should not be exactly perpendicular to the ear, but should stand at about a 20-degree angle. This will keep any melting wax that runs down the inside of the candle from depositing in the ear, and will help to keep the tip clear of hardened wax. If smoke is escaping from the ear, please set the candle again.

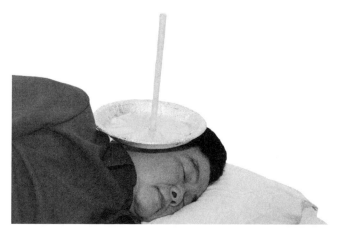

Fig. 3.16. Ear candling

4. After the first 2 minutes, remove the candle from the ear and clean out the tip with a toothpick. This will keep smoke flowing into the ear canal.

5. Remove the candle from the ear about every 3 minutes. Check to see that the tip is open, and trim off the burned portion of the candle into the bowl of water with a sharp pair of scissors. This will maximize the amount of smoke going into the ear, though you should be careful not to trim away so much that the flame is extinguished.

6. Do not let the candle burn down to less than 3" from the end. When you are done, extinguish the burning end in the bowl of water and dispose of it in a safe manner. At this time, you may choose to place 1 or 2 drops of an unrefined oil (like sunflower, sesame, or olive oil) into the ear openings to loosen up any remaining wax, thereby improving the hearing.

For best results, the candler should massage gently around the ears and eyes during candling process. This will help to release any blockages.

Chi Self-Massage Ear Exercises

Outer Ear, Ear Shells, Earlobes

Contract the left and right sides of the anus while rubbing your hands together vigorously. Bring accumulated energy into your hands.

1. **Front and back:** Make a space between your index and ring fingers and simultaneously rub the front and back of the ears.
2. **Ear shells:** Rub the ear shells with all of your fingers. This will stimulate the autonomic nervous system and warm up your whole body, especially in the cold weather.
3. **Earlobes:** Using your thumb and index finger, gently pull down on the earlobes (fig. 3.17).

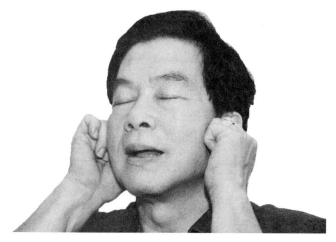

Fig. 3.17. Earlobe pulling

☯ *Eardrums*

Bring energy to the hands while contracting the left and right sides of anus.

1. Inhale and then exhale completely.
2. Put your index fingers into your ears (fig. 3.18); it should feel as if there is a vacuum in the ears. If it does not, then exhale more.

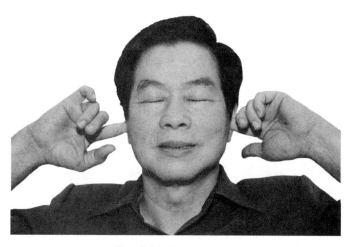

Fig. 3.18. Ear popping

3. Move your index fingers back and forth 6 to 9 times at your own pace until you can feel that the insides of the ears are moving, then pull out the fingers with a quick movement. You should hear a "pop" sound, and you will feel that you can hear better and that your mind is clearer.

☯ Inner Ear

Bring energy to the hands while contracting the left and right sides of the anus.

Because it is inaccessible, the inner ear is not usually exercised and it grows weaker with age. However, the following two exercises use air pressure and vibration to strengthen the inner ear. By building up pressure inside of the lungs, mouth, and nose canal, we can add pressure to the inner ear and exercise it in this way.

O Blowing Exercise

1. Inhale through the nose, filling your lungs and nasal cavity with air. Then close your mouth and pinch your nostrils shut with your index finger and thumb.
2. Blow slowly outward toward your closed nostrils, and then swallow air. You should feel your eardrums popping.
3. Repeat two to three times.

Do not blow too hard as your eardrums can get hurt. You must do every exercise gently for the most benefit.

O Ear and Nervous System Exercise — Hitting the Eardrum

1. Cover your ears with your palms, fingers pointing toward the back of your head.

2. In this position, flick your index finger against the third finger so that the index fingers drum on the occipital bone, which forms the lower edge of the skull (fig. 3.19). This will sound quite loud. The finger hitting the bone will create a vibration that stimulates the nervous system, the ears, and the mechanisms of the inner ears.

3. Repeat 9 times or more. The activity of the ear will be balanced and the mastoid sinus improved by this exercise.

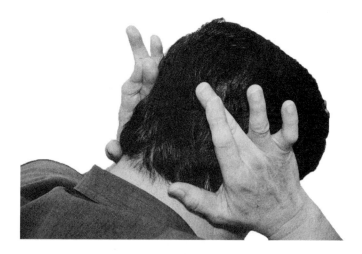

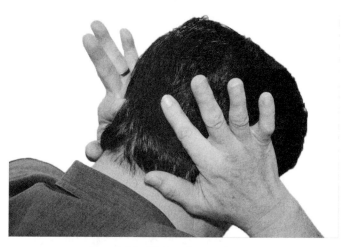

Fig. 3.19. Hitting the eardrum

THE MOUTH

The mouth is the window of communication and love in the universe. To maintain the opening of the mouth in good condition, the Taoists recommend the regular practice of mouth exercises and tongue scraping, and periodic cleanses using unrefined vegetable oil.

The opening of the mouth also includes the lips, gums, tongue, throat, teeth, heart, and spleen/pancreas. For this reason, all of the exercises for taking care of the mouth will also benefit these organs and tissues. They will strengthen both the gums and teeth, for instance, which will improve bad breath and build the strength of the bones.

Because saliva is an essential form of energy that lubricates the organs and digestive system, several of the exercises make use of saliva to activate body cleansing processes (fig. 3.20).

The tongue is the opening of the heart, and both are made of similar tissue. A healthy and clean tongue will strengthen the organs, especially the heart. You should clean your tongue twice a day with a brush or scrape it with a tongue scraper, and massage your tongue with a tongue depressor or a clean finger. Find the painful spots and massage there until the pain goes away. This mouth cleanse will activate, cleanse, and refresh your mouth, tongue, teeth and gums.

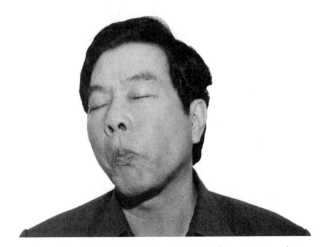

Fig. 3.20. Clean the mouth with saliva and swallow it several times.

Oil Mouth Cleanse for the Spleen and Stomach

Oil therapy is a simple, yet astoundingly effective method of cleansing the blood, gums, teeth, and mouth.* It can improve numerous disorders including blood diseases, lung and liver disorders, tooth and gum diseases, headaches, skin diseases, gastric ulcers, intestinal problems, poor appetite, heart/kidney ailments, encephalitis, nervous conditions, poor memory, female disorders, swollen face, and bags under the eyes.

For this cleanse you will need the following ingredients:

1 teaspoon cold-pressed, unrefined sunflower, sesame, or
   olive oil
½ teaspoon baking soda or unrefined sea salt
1 teaspoon hydrogen peroxide

1. On an empty stomach, slowly swish the oil in your mouth. Chew it, swirl it around, and draw it through your teeth for 3 to 4 minutes. This thoroughly mixes the oil with saliva, releasing and activating enzymes that then draw toxins out of the blood.
2. Spit out the oil after no more than 3 to 4 minutes. This will keep the released toxins from being reabsorbed. You will find that the oil takes on a milky white or yellowish color as it becomes saturated with toxins and billions of destructive bacteria.
3. For best results, repeat this process 2 more times.
4. Dissolve ½ teaspoon of baking soda or ½ teaspoon unrefined sea salt in a small amount of water and rinse out your mouth with this solution. It will remove all remnants of the oil and toxins. Additionally, you may want to brush your teeth and scrape your tongue to make sure your mouth is clean (see fig. 3.21 on page 76).

---

*This recipe is from Andreas Moritz, *The Liver and Gallbladder Miracle Cleanse* (Berkeley, Calif.: Ulysses Press, 2007).

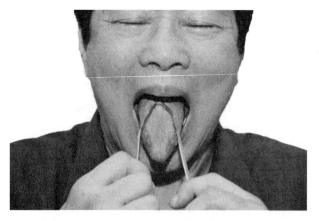

Fig. 3.21. Tongue scraping

Some visible effects of oil swishing include the elimination of gum bleeding and the whitening of teeth. During times of illness, this procedure can be repeated 3 times per day, but only on an empty stomach. Oil therapy greatly relieves and supports liver functions, as it takes toxins out of the blood that the liver has not been able to remove or detoxify. This benefits the entire organism.

Chi Self-Massage Mouth Exercises

Gums

Open your mouth and stretch your lips tautly over your teeth. Use three fingertips (index, middle, and ring fingers) to tap the skin around upper and lower gums. Hit around until you feel warmth in the area. These exercises will help to improve foul breath and to clarify speech.

Gums and Tongue

1. Massage your upper and lower gums with your tongue (fig. 3.22).
2. Suck in some saliva and press your tongue tightly against the roof of your mouth. Press around. When you strengthen your tongue, you are strengthening your heart. Press the tongue to the roof of

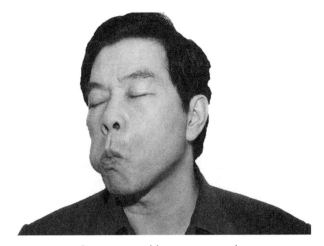

Fig. 3.22. Massage the upper and lower gums with your tongue.

your mouth, tighten your neck muscles and swallow the saliva. This lubricates the digestive glands and organs.

⚙ Tongue

1. In a sitting position, place your hands on your knees, palms down. Exhale and straighten your arms keeping your hands on your knees and spreading the fingers apart.
2. Still exhaling, open your mouth as wide as possible and thrust your tongue out and down, focusing on the throat (see fig. 3.23 on page 78).
3. With your tongue out as far possible, gaze at the tip of your nose and tense up your whole body. Hold your breath for as long as you feel comfortable.
4. Relax with inhalation and regulate your breath. This will help to strengthen the throat, the tongue, and the power of speech.
5. Inhale, then exhale as you press your tongue out and down again as far as you can.
6. Follow by pulling your tongue in and curling it. Press your tongue to the roof of your mouth as hard as you can, contracting the middle of the anus and the esophagus to help the tongue.

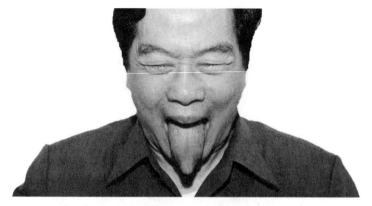

Fig. 3.23. Thrust your tongue out and down as far as possible.

With more practice you will know how to use the inside force, the force from the organs, to press your tongue up. Even though the tongue has no bones to exert force, you will still be able to exercise the tongue well.

Teeth Clenching and Energizing

1. Relax your lips. Click your teeth together lightly and then clench them hard (fig. 3.24) as you inhale and pull up the middle of the anus. Do this 6 to 9 times.
2. Move your tongue and mouth to create a lot of saliva. The best technique for swallowing saliva is to put your tongue up to your palate and then swallow quickly with a hard gulp, sending the saliva down the esophagus to your stomach.
3. Close your mouth and let your teeth touch lightly. Direct your energy to your teeth, and gradually feel the electrical flow of energy there.

Stomach-Acid Cleanse

The modern acidic diet often causes the stomach to become overloaded with acid, resulting in heartburn, stomach pain, and bloating.

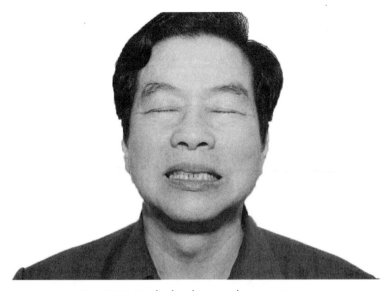

Fig. 3.24. Teeth clenching and energizing

This is a simple cleanse that can be very effective at reducing excess acidity in the stomach.

1. Mix 1 teaspoon baking soda (sodium bicarbonate) in 8 ounces of warm water.
2. Slowly swish this solution in your mouth, chewing it and drawing it through your teeth for 3 to 4 minutes. Then swallow it.

THE NOSTRILS

The nostrils are the window of life and higher consciousness. To maintain them in good health, the Taoists recommend regular practice of chi self-massage nose exercises, along with periodic nasal washes and nasal rubs.

The opening of the nostrils includes the nose, sinuses, diaphragm, and lungs, such that the exercises and cleanses described below will benefit all of these organs and tissues. Conversely, any exercises that strengthen the lungs and/or diaphragm will also strengthen the opening of the nose.

Nasal Douching

You will need 1 teaspoon of sea salt dissolved in 8 ounces warm water, a plastic nasal douching bottle or a neti pot, and eucalyptus oil—1 drop for each nostril.

1. Using the plastic bottle or neti pot, insert the warm water and salt solution into one nostril. Pass it around through the sinuses and out the other nostril (fig. 3.25). This will begin to break up any debris in the nasal passages.

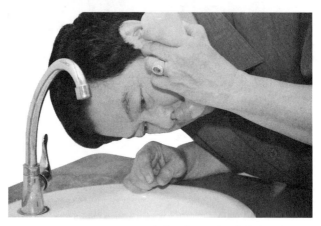

Fig. 3.25. Nasal-douching cleanse

2. To activate, stimulate, and heal these passages after washing them as described above, rub 1 drop of eucalyptus oil into the nasal passage of each nostril.

 ## Chi Self-Massage Nose Exercises

Nostrils

Widen the nostrils. Stick the thumb and index finger of either hand into the nostrils and move them to the left and right, and up and down 10 to 20 times (fig. 3.26). This will increase the passage of air into the lungs, improving any sinus problems and the sense of smell.

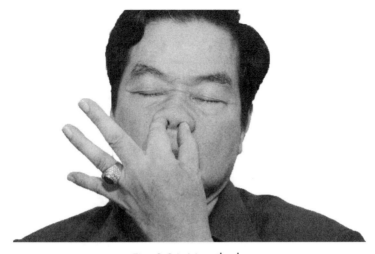

Fig. 3.26. Nostril rub

Nose Bridge

Massage the bridge of your nose by repeatedly pinching it with your thumb and index finger (fig. 3.27). As you do this, inhale slowly and imagine you are breathing in clean air; exhale slowly and imagine you are exhaling dirty air. Do this 9 to 36 times. This is effective for blocked sinuses.

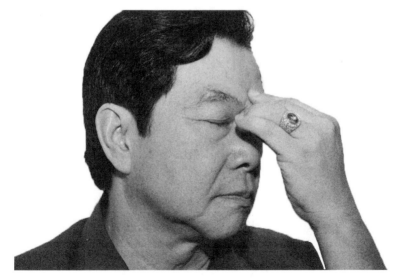

Fig. 3.27. Nose-bridge massage

🌀 Mid-Nose

For the mid-nose, place your thumb and third finger or either side of your nose, on the bone just before it turns into cartilage (fig 3.28). Place your index finger on the bridge, inhale, and press in gently. Then exhale and relax. Feel the heat in your fingers and absorb it into your nose. This exercise can increase your concentration and calm your mind.

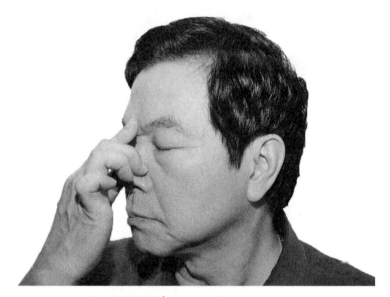

Fig. 3.28. Mid-nose massage

🌀 Sides of the Nose

Use your two index fingers to slowly massage up and down the sides of your nose 9 to 36 times (fig. 3.29). Rub the sides of your nose up and down until you feel warm, but begin with light pressure and increase it slowly, because the tissues there are very tender and easily infected.

This exercise will help to release blocked sinuses and stuffy noses. It will also help you in the cold winter and every morning when you get up.

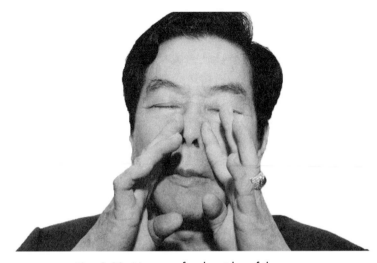

Fig. 3.29. Massage for the sides of the nose

🌀 Lower Nose

To massage the lower end of your nose, place your index finger immediately under the nose, at a right angle to it (fig. 3.30). Massage slowly at first; then gradually increase to a vigorous back-and-forth massage when you are sure that you will not hurt yourself. This exercise helps blocked sinuses and stuffy, runny noses.

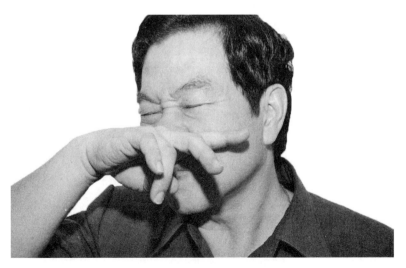

Fig. 3.30. Lower nose massage

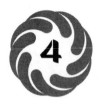

Other Natural Therapies

This chapter explores the notion of cleansing right down to the level of individual cells. The health of your cells is a direct expression of what you are absorbing into your body. From a macroscopic perspective, it is hard to imagine what is happening on the cellular level, but we have many modern tools to verify what ancient wisdom has always told us about our bodies: our cells are responsible for carrying and storing nutrients, organisms, and waste, but they can also incubate disease, viruses, and bacteria. For this reason, it is important to clean them out regularly.

Focusing on cells gives an interesting insight into the dynamic nature of the human body. Because the number of cells in your body is continually changing as old cells die and new ones are replicated, your whole body is in a state of flux; dynamic events are happening right now, in every moment of every day. From this perspective, what is health really? It is the unobstructed functioning of the individual cells within your body.

As you go through your day, your body reacts to all the materials thrown at it in the form of food, radiation, pressure, temperature, etc. These energy dynamics put stress on the system, which can then become congested in a variety of ways and lead to illness or disease. As noted in previous chapters, the degree to which you are able to move things through your body, or get them unstuck, determines the level of health you can enjoy.

One might ask, how can I clean out the insides of my cells? In fact, what this chapter explains is how to remove the unwanted material *in between* the trillions of cells in your body, so that they can accomplish their work. You will journey through different natural methods of cleaning out the intercellular spaces of your body via the blood, the colon, and the energy fields of your cells in order to maximize their receptivity to the divine forces at work every day in our universe.

COLLOIDAL SILVER

Silver has benefited mankind's health for thousands of years. In ancient Greece and Rome, people used silver containers to keep liquids fresh. American settlers traveling across the West often put a silver dollar in their milk to delay its spoiling. Around the turn of the century, doctors prescribed silver nitrate for stomach ulcers and it has been a common practice to put a few drops of a silver solution in newborn babies' eyes to kill bacteria that causes blindness.

Normally, we obtain silver and all other minerals in our bodies through the foods we eat. They come directly from organic soil, which is rich in living organisms. These organisms break the soil down so that plants can assimilate the minerals from it. However, if we eat plants that have been grown with chemical insecticides and fertilizers, as most plants are today, the soil—and thus the plants—will be lacking many of the vitamins and minerals that are available in foods grown in healthy, living soils. This is how deficiencies develop in our modern food supplies.

As the body tissues age, or if we cannot assimilate silver for some other reason, we develop a silver deficiency and an impaired immune system that can lead to cancer and other diseases. Some suspect that silver deficiency is one of the main reasons cancer is increasing at such a rapid rate today. Dr. Robert O. Becker, M.D., orthopedic surgeon and medical research doctor, noticed a correlation between low silver levels and sickness. People who had low silver levels were frequently sick, with innumerable colds, flu, fevers, and other illnesses. He suggested that silver deficiency prevented the immune system from functioning properly. He found that supplemental silver works against a wide range of bacteria and can stimulate major growth of injured tissues, without any side effects or damage to the body cells.

Colloidal silver is a pure, all-natural substance consisting of sub-microscopic clusters of silver, held in a suspension of pure ionized water by a tiny electric charge placed on each particle. Advocates of colloidal silver know that it is a powerful antiviral agent and bactericide, as well as a fever reducer. It can be helpful in the treatment of infections following childbirth, cystitis, staph infections, septicemia, pneumonia, flu, and even cancer, among other ailments. However, it has a somewhat checkered reputation in the medical world, such that reliable information about this valuable supplement can be difficult to find.

An easily assimilable form of silver that has many medical uses *and* some controversy around it, colloidal silver is the subject of countless medical journal reports. It has been found to be both a remedy and a prevention for colds, flu, and other infections or fermentations due to any bacteria, fungus, or virus. It is even effective against staphylococcus and streptococcus infections, which are often found in diseased conditions. It has been reported to rapidly subdue inflammation and promote faster healing. Whereas any particular pharmaceutical antibiotic kills, on average, six different disease organisms, colloidal silver is known to kill over 650 diseases without any known harmful side effects or toxicity. Taken daily, colloidal silver provides a second immune system resulting in more energy, vitality, vigor, relaxation, faster healing, and reduced bodily toxins.

Colloidal silver is odorless, tasteless, nonstinging, harmless to eyes, contains no free radicals, is harmless to human enzymes, and has no reaction with other medications. It improves digestion, causes rapid regeneration of damaged cells and tissues, helps prevent colds, flu, and all organism-caused diseases.

Unfortunately, commercial production of silver products is not regulated by any agency, so there are wide variations in the quality of "colloidal" silver products. In fact, there are three distinctly different types of silver that are labeled and sold on the market as "colloidal silver"—they are ionic silver, silver protein, and true colloidal silver. Consumers seeking true colloidal silver are often at a disadvantage because each of these products represents themselves as colloidal silver.

In true colloidal silver, the majority of the silver content is in the form of silver particles. True colloids will typically contain 50–80 percent silver particles, with the balance being silver ions. True colloidal silver is nontoxic, nonaddictive, and has no known side effects. The body develops no tolerance and one cannot overdose. It cannot cause harm to liver, kidneys, organs, or any part of the body, and is safe for pregnant and nursing women, even aiding the developing fetus in growth and health, as well as easing the mother's delivery and recovery.

Due to the very low concentration of ionic silver and small particle size, true silver colloids do not cause *argyria*, a condition that causes the skin to permanently turn blue-gray. However, silver protein preparations—which are not true colloids, though they are often labeled as such—*can* cause argyria, and there are a few documented cases of it in the medical research. Because of these isolated incidents, the medical establishment is extremely leery of silver supplementation, and most medical associations and agencies, including the FDA, have deemed it "not safe and effective." Dr. Becker's conclusion is that while there is not enough research submitted to substantively prove the medical benefits of colloidal silver, there is certainly no evidence to prove it is dangerous.

It is easy to see why colloidal silver is not distributed in the general marketplace as much as it could be—because there is no way to verify the efficacy of a substance labeled "colloidal silver" on the shelves of our drug stores and pharmacies. Naturally, the FDA cannot support such a substance if it has no way to control the quality of the product it endorses. Indeed, you should shy away from any untrusted sources or unsubstantiated claims that a substance is indeed colloidal silver if you attempt to obtain some for yourself. In the resources section on page 151, you can find some resources for information about colloidal silver, and places to purchase it.

ENERGIZED WATER

Who are the oldest and healthiest people on the planet? They live in Hunza Valley in Northeast Pakistan. Cancer, tooth decay, high blood pressure, just about all of the top killers in the world today really are not found in the people of Hunza Valley. Why? They have no GNC, they do not take vitamins, supplements, or exotic juices; they just eat regular villager food and drink lots of water. While the average apricot tree lives 25–30 years, apricot trees in Hunza Valley live well past 100 years old.

The Hunza Valley is a real place, and its health is in the water. That is it, just plain and simple water. The key is they are drinking very old, protected water from an ancient glacier. It has not been exposed to all the pollution that water in the rest of the world has. Hunza water emits a frequency at 80 Hertz, meaning it has very small cluster sizes. Average tap water and even very expensive Evian water are at 120 Hertz, indicating very large cluster sizes. So large, in fact, that the average person in the world is dehydrated by the time they are 30 years old because the water they drink is too big to penetrate into the cells. The water in Hunza Valley is also quite soft, with a low surface tension that allows it to get into your cells and hydrate them very well, unlike hard water.

Japanese and European scientists have long known that there are natural pools of energized waters similar to Hunza valley water deep in the Earth's core, some hundreds to thousands of meters deep. These types of very pure energized waters pulsate at a unique frequency of around 53–62 Hertz. These natural energized waters have been used in Japan and Europe since ancient times for therapeutic spas, food preservation, and beer production, among other applications.

On the other hand, scientists using resonance tests prove that most of today's tap water, distilled water, and spring/mountain waters resonate at 120 to 130 Hertz, demonstrating that they are quite removed from their original, pure state. This is what has happened to our everyday water, slowly eroded by acid rain and the pollution from industrial and agricultural chemicals.

Today, energized water from these natural pools can be purchased, but it is cost-prohibitive because of expensive sourcing costs. Instead, it is possible to revitalize or energize regular water, and thereby return it to its natural state.

The science behind energized water may seem magical but it is not; it is linked to the physics of water—its vibrational resonance—rather than its chemistry. The differences can be scientifically measured. For instance, the molecular clusters of energized water are smaller (i.e., nano-sized), and they vibrate faster. Such waters have much lower surface tension, and are able to inhibit bacteria, reduce odors, neutralize chlorine smells, retain food freshness longer, inhibit oxidation better, remove rust and corrosion faster, and even taste better.

In *The Healing Power of Energized Water*, author Ulrich Holst outlines the properties of water that make it possible to revitalize water that has been stripped of its dynamic energetic properties.

1. As water is a highly sensitive substance, it reacts immediately to outside influences, both positively and negatively. These reactions include its ability to restructure itself on a molecular level, an increase or reduction of its vitality (photon emission), and its memory, depending on how it is imprinted or revitalized.
2. Healthy, vital water is able to process impurities, pollutants, and stress—in other words, it has the ability to regenerate. This

regeneration is connected to its swirling movement, its natural spiral coiling (implosion). Similarly, it has the ability to assimilate negative information—at least up to a certain point.

3. When polluted water is put in contact with a spring or another form of concentrated vital energy (chi, orgone, tachyons, and so on) that is harmoniously structured on the subatomic level, not only will it revitalize but it will also recover its innate power to purify and heal, by virtue of the biocatalytic process.

4. Many procedures and techniques have been developed over the last several decades for producing concentrated forms of bioenergy and transmitting it to devitalized—dirty or polluted—water.

5. Revitalized water that has been redynamized on the molecular level recovers its innate ability to absorb oxygen and loses surface tension. It therefore becomes softer and more fluid. The minerals that remain suspended in such water and make it hard are carried away in the water instead of being deposited on the walls of blood vessels or water pipes.

Furthermore, biologically healthy water:

• More easily rids itself of impurities (meaning fewer cleaning products are needed).
• Is better at eliminating wastes from the human body.
• Is a better bonding agent in production of cement, paint, and so forth.
• More readily absorbs oxygen, nutritive substances, and minerals.
• Encourages the germination of plants.
• Helps to preserve cut flowers, and fresh fruits and vegetables.
• Is a superior conductor of heat (thus reducing the energy needed in water-based heating systems).*

---

*Ulrich Holst, *The Healing Power of Energized Water* (Rochester, Vt.: Healing Arts Press, 2010.

Dr. Albert Einstein once profoundly stated that everything in life is vibration. Modern science, using magnetic resonance imaging equipment, contends that every existing thing in this universe emits a unique frequency that affects not only its surrounding environment, but even objects at great distances. The speed of sound in water travels nearly four times faster than the speed of sound in air (1500 meters per second versus 400 mps). Do you recall the violent force of the tsunami off the Indonesian coast? This force (measured as energy or frequency) traveled an astonishing 1,200 miles across the Indian Ocean in three hours—as fast as an airliner traveling underwater—but if you were sitting in a boat in the middle of the ocean, you could barely feel this incredible vibrating energy passing under you.

Another phenomenon of vibration science is utilized in the 2,300-year-old practice of Traditional Chinese acupuncture, which uses frequency (conducted via movements of the needles) to stimulate our health. Pressure (think in terms of frequency) exerted at precise acupuncture points sends an energy signal into our tissue cells, organs, diseases, toxins, and microbes, and when these frequencies (energies) are balanced, our diseases are relieved. Other forms of healing that make active use of vibrational energy are acupressure, Reiki, homeopathy, magnetic healing, aromatherapy, and gem therapy, among others. In modern medicine, we use the vibrational attributes of magnets to create MRI images and sound vibrations to create sonograms. Vibrational frequencies are used in other branches of science to measure objects under water and in space.

About 15 years ago, the Japanese discovered revolutionary techniques to produce energized water by passing water simultaneously over an electromagnetic rod and kiln-fired ceramic mineral stones. This phenomenon allows regular tap water to change its frequency to below 80 Hertz. As our Earth's environment continuously deteriorates, there is greater demand for improved bio and eco balance and the use of energized water provides a revolutionary solution to these problems.

Today, there are many different products available that energize water by various means. Some use permanent magnets, others use crystals, swirling motions, vibrations, or subatomic energies like tachyons. What all of these methods have in common is the notion that devitalized water can be healed, and that plants, animals, and people will benefit from better water. Indeed, researchers studying the effects of energized water have noted that it is better than regular water at eliminating wastes from the human body, that it more readily absorbs oxygen, minerals, and nutrients from food and the environment, and that it cleans dirt and impurities more effectively than regular water, requiring less soap and cleansers during clean-up jobs. In addition, energized water encourages the germination and growth of plants and preserves cut flowers for much longer than regular water.

All of this information adds up to the simple conclusion that energized, re-dynamized water is an important component of health for all living things. To begin your own rediscovery of water, see our resources section on pages 151–52.

FASTING (WATER ONLY)

There are many types of fasts that can be undertaken to cleanse and purify your organs. You can do 2–3-day fasts on certain whole foods to cleanse and flush out specific organs such as the heart (steamed kale), kidneys (watermelon), lungs (steamed garlic and dandelion greens), spleen (steamed yellow/orange tubers), and liver (apple juice). Or you can fast on water only, giving your body one day a week or one weekend a month to rest the digestive system and rejuvenate itself.

On a water fast, you allow the body to break down excess debris, so it can open up and free itself. The less you do the better; this is the fine art of fasting. In other words, you lie down and relax doing nothing, which is the hardest thing for our monkey minds to do. You may do a little bit of reading, but it's better to mostly just observe and drink water to hydrate yourself. This will flush the body, allowing your urine to take out the debris; you literally urinate yourself back to health. Initially there will be foul odor from the urine, but after a while there will be no smell at all.

When you get a disease in the body, your body is telling you to stop doing what you've been doing, and that means stop eating and refrain from any excess activities. This allows the energy that would be expended to digest the food or surf the Internet to be utilized in breaking down any blockages. This is the cheapest and easiest way to approach the problem of disease.

Standard medical practice in the West tends to eliminate blockages by eliminating (via surgery) those parts of the body that are suffering from them. This is fine except that when an organ has been surgically removed, you lose its function. When you have a blockage in the body, the easiest way to solve the problem is to allow the body to eliminate the blockage itself. To summon the added energy required to do this, you simply take energy away from the digesting and thinking processes.

You are in an inactive state when you do this kind of fasting (fig. 4.1). It is amazing that people have very little time to do nothing because they are so busy doing everything. They try to find solutions where the solution is so simple that they cannot see it. Taoist meditative practices, on the other hand, allow the mind to slow down, so that everything becomes clear to you—including what to do by non-doing.

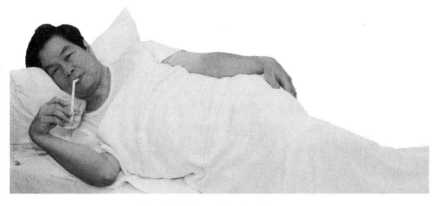

Fig. 4.1. Water-fasting therapy

You start to make some conscious choices instead of simply reacting, resulting in proper and correct action. This is called Wu Wei, the art of doing absolutely nothing.

FRUITARIANISM

Through the carnivorous diet accepted by man during the past centuries came the lowest physical form of living—actually killing and eating our earthly coinhabitants. Yet nature will not tolerate persistent, continuous abuse without exacting a penalty: the illnesses we suffer are a direct result of our gluttonous, denatured diets. Still, the process of transitioning to a fruitarian diet is not for everyone. Only the inspired person can understand the fruitarian preference, which is the food of nature. We live in an age when man is in open rebellion against nature, which probably means that only a chosen few will listen and reap the benefits of nature's teachings.

The simple truth of present times is more difficult to believe than the wildest fiction: hundreds of millions of humans throughout the civilized world today are depleted in vitality and live only half-useful lives. Neither religion nor a university education can create vibrant health and radiant vitality. You can regain and retain health through a mucus-free diet consisting of fruits and starchless vegetables, exercise, breathing, walks, and proper daily choices (i.e., fresh air, sunlight, and pure water)! These are the curative agents. Allow nature, in her own way, to repair and restore the ravages of disease, slowly but surely.

KOMBUCHA TEA

Kombucha tea is made by adding a colony of bacteria and yeast (often referred to as a "mushroom,") to sugar and black tea, and allowing them to ferment. Health benefits attributed to Kombucha tea include stimulating the immune system, preventing cancer, and improving digestion and liver function.

Kombucha tea is commonly prepared by taking a starter sample from an existing culture (the "Mother" mushroom) and growing a new colony in a fresh jar. You can buy premade kombucha in many health food stores, or you can brew your own. For information on where to obtain a starter culture and other supplies, see the resources section on page 152.

Kombucha Tea Recipe

Upon receipt of your starter culture, allow air to enter the bag(s) before refrigerating; start your first batch of tea within 3–4 days.

1. Fill a pan (preferably an enamel or porcelain pan) with 3½ quarts of good quality water.
2. Bring water almost to a boil and add 1 cup of white sugar (preferably sugar cane derived sugar rather than sugar beet sugar), and 10 drops of "racemized" sea minerals if you have them.
3. Stir, remove from heat, and add 5 bags of regular black tea or Chinese tea (Lipton or Red Rose orange pekoe/pekoe cut teas are fine, but don't use instant or herbal teas, or green teas).
4. Steep for 10–15 minutes; remove bags, let cool to room temperature.
5. Next, pour solution into a one gallon wide-mouthed glass jar (look for old pickle or mayonnaise jars from restaurants), or into a porcelain enamel pan, a glazed crock, or a plastic container like a water pitcher or Tupperware.
6. Add starter tea inoculant and mushroom from starter bag or from last batch. (The murky tea in the bottom of each batch contains "spores" and makes the best inoculant.) Cover container with a paper napkin or paper towel (don't use cloth material), and secure the cover with a rubber band.
7. Incubate this tea at room temperature for 14 days. Adjust incubation time based on room temperature (longer for cooler weather, shorter in summer) in order to produce a tea that is more vinegary than sweet. Shorter duration batches taste better, but do not have the ability to rejuvenate the body.

8. Each new batch produces a baby bacterial colony that begins to form on about day eight (look for a thin membrane or scummy film forming above the mother on the surface equal to the diameter of the container. The mother grows darker with age, while the offspring will be more translucent in appearance and will form whitish spots as it matures and may have darkish spots of tea lignins (brown pigments) on underside of mushroom.

9. Drink each batch within 72 hours: 3 mugs a day.

Limit initial Kombucha consumption to ½ cup the first day or two. Increase consumption over several days. Kombucha is a very powerful, whole body rejuvenator and should be taken between meals on an empty stomach. If your system reacts too severely, adjust your intake for a short time. Kombucha tea is a powerful tissue cleanser.

When starting a new batch, repeat the above process. Sometimes you have to divide mother and baby mushrooms by peeling them apart (layers meld and can become very thick and fibrous if left for several batches making it difficult to separate them). If you tear a hole in your baby, it will not do any harm.

Note: Never make or store tea in a metal container, especially aluminum. Keep finished tea refrigerated in glass or plastic. The mushroom is not eaten. Never let the mushroom remain in contact with metal or it will die. The mushroom is a living chemical factory. It converts left-spin energy (white sugar) into a right-spin energy (energy is never lost, it merely changes form). The tea is loaded with enzymes, organic acids, hormones, and vitamins. Do not substitute honey, fructose, turbinado sugar, or brown sugars for the "evil" white sugar. Use common tea-bag tea. Keep it simple, have fun.

✪ Keeping a Permanent Brew

1. Start your own "mother" mushroom with the starter tea you receive and transfer some from a previous batch each and every time.

2. Space batches about 3 days apart until you have as many batches "brewing" as needed to meet your needs. When on vacation, incubate a batch for up to 45 days. Upon return, use sediment in bottom of batch to "start" several batches at once to get your routine going again.

3. Throw away the mother mushroom every second batch or when it becomes too thick, and substitute with the baby. Mushrooms have personalities. Some sink, some float; some batches of tea are carbonated, others not; most mothers produce babies, some don't. Just go with the flow and don't freak out.

MONO-DIET CLEANSING

Mono-diet cleansing allows you to reap many of the benefits of fasting while still eating some solid food every day. By restricting your food intake to only one kind of fruit or vegetable for a few days, you allow your body to absorb vitamins and minerals while it cleanses itself of many built-up toxins (fig. 4.2).

The following fruits can be used in a mono-diet cleanse for 3–10 days with maxumium benefits for digestion, skin, organ function, hair, and nails.

Avocados

The avocado is a highly nutritious fruit that has a relatively high fat content. Avocados (*Persea americana*) were first cultivated in South and Central America, and were a staple in the Aztec diet.

Avocados are a good source of potassium, containing more than twice as much potassium as bananas. They are also rich in protein, beta-carotene, vitamin B complex, vitamin E, lecithin, fluorine, and copper. Avocados are cooling and especially beneficial for dry skin and hair. They strengthen the blood, and have traditionally been recommended for erectile dysfunction, nervousness, and insomnia. They are also nourishing during convalescence.

Banana

Botanists have placed the cultivation of the banana in the Indus Valley around 2000 BCE. Early peoples domesticated the fruit from the wild variety during that period. Bananas stimulate the production of serotonin, a compound that can improve sleep and elevate mood. They are high in calories but low in fat. As for nutritional sufficiency, bananas are at the top of the list. Rich in carbohydrates, folic acid, B_6, and vitamin C, bananas provide long-term energy and stamina, and moisten the yin fluids of the body. Six pounds of bananas will supply about 2,380 calories.

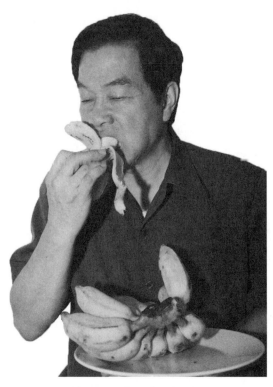

Fig. 4.2. Mono-fruit diet therapy

Figs

Syrian figs (*Ficus curica*) are one of the earliest fruits cultivated by man. They were grown as early as 4000 BCE. and spread all over the eastern Mediterranean region centuries ago. Figs are warming and alkaline in nature. They are rich in vitamin B6, folic acid, calcium, copper, iron, magnesium, manganese, phosphorus, and potassium. Figs are said to improve energy levels, and to boost fertility.

Mango

Mangos (*Mangifera indica*) were first cultivated in India over 2,000 years ago. Akbar, the Mogul emperor of India during the sixteenth century, so loved the mango that he planted an orchard of 100,000 mango trees.

Mangos are cooling and tonic to the yin organs, providing moistening fluids for the body. They have been traditionally used to treat anemia, calm the emotions, benefit the brain, strengthen the heart, and provide energy. Mangoes are rich in beta-carotene, niacin, vitamin C, flavonoids, vitamin E, iron, and potassium.

Tomatoes

Tomatoes originated in South America in what is now Peru. They are powerful immune system boosters, and are even thought to help prevent many cancers. Tomatoes are rich in vitamin A, thiamine, riboflavin, and vitamin C. A raw tomato is about 90 percent water. A 3½-ounce tomato has 24 calories, about 1 percent protein and about 4 percent carbohydrate.

SEAWATER

The seawater cleanse is a technique used by many island cultures to reverse the effects of aging, heal the body, and renew vitality and energy. The cleanse is relatively simple but very powerful. Every day you drink a hyper-tonic fluid (salt water), which pulls fluid into your intestine and causes diarrhea. Most people have a backlog of poop so they will need to defecate 2–4 times per day. It's important to drink a lot of regular water throughout the day.

 ## Seawater Cleanse

If you have problems with constipation, please clean your bowels with a safe herbal laxative (senna or garcinia) for one or two days before this cleanse.

Avoid alcohol, spicy foods, fried foods, and anything rich or heavy during this week of cleansing. You will take your digestive tract back to its childhood state. Think of what would be best to feed a small child and you will know what to eat.

Beginning the Cleanse

Do the following for 5–10 days.

1. **6:00 a.m.** Drink 1 gallon of heated seawater (fig. 4.3).
2. **9:00 a.m.** Drink 1 quart of vegetable juice (shake).
3. **12:00 p.m.** Drink 1 quart of fruit juice (shake).
4. **5:00 p.m.** Drink 2 bowls of vegetable broth.

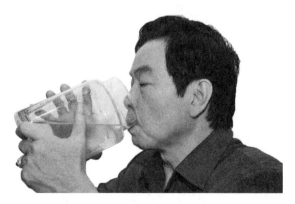

Fig. 4.3. Seawater therapy

☯ Final Two Days

1. **6:00 a.m.** Drink 1 gallon of heated seawater.
2. Eat normally—fruits and vegetables first, then more complex carbohydrates (starches) and proteins (animal products) gradually.

URINE THERAPY

The use of urine for healing has a history that goes back thousands of years. Medical manuals from ancient Egypt devote hundreds of pages to urine therapy, while in the West, it was Hippocrates who first cataloged and promoted the benefits of urine as medicine. Because our modern culture disdains all discussion of waste and waste products, most people today have never even heard of urine therapy; those who have usually find the idea bizarre, if not completely repulsive. The Taoists, however, have long recognized urine therapy as a simple, effective remedy for a variety of ills.

When applied externally to wounds, rashes, or other skin conditions, urine provides a fast, safe method of healing. It also has many cosmetic uses and can be used in massage lotions. However, the greatest benefits of urine therapy come from drinking it. A small amount of morning urine drunk daily can safely heal the body from bacterial illnesses, inflammatory ailments, and can even improve severe illnesses like cancer and autoimmune disease.

Although many people are uncomfortable with the idea of ingesting urine, it is important to remember that our urine is not just waste. It contains valuable hormones, neurotransmitters, and immune system cells that the body felt a need to release to combat infections, diseases, allergies, and other disturbances. When we drink our urine, we confront our immune systems with this information for a second time, allowing it to mount a second, more effective defense.

Urine Therapy Basics

A clean glass or clear plastic container is best for collecting urine. In research studies, urine is usually collected by means of a "clean catch," in which the genital area is cleansed before collecting the urine and only midstream urine is collected. This is particularly important for women using urine therapy internally; it can be done by simply washing with a little soap and water.

Collect the midstream urine by urinating for a second or two without collecting anything, then urinating into your container. Stop when the container is almost full, and empty whatever is left in your bladder into the toilet. The midstream urine is the only urine you should use, as it contains the nutrients and immune system information you need, without any impurities that may be cleaned out by the beginning and end of the stream.

Urine breaks down quickly outside the body so use it internally within fifteen minutes of collection. If you are going to use it for external use only, this isn't as important, and you can use either fresh urine or urine that has been stored for a day or two.

Urine Therapy—External Uses

◌ *Treating Skin Disorders*

Applying urine to the skin is an excellent treatment for every imaginable type of skin disorder, including all rashes, eczema, psoriasis, and acne.

1. Use either fresh or old urine for skin applications, although old urine has a higher ammonia content and has been found to be more effective in treating many stubborn skin disorders such as eczema or psoriasis.
2. Pour a small amount of urine onto a cotton ball or pad and pat or massage it lightly onto the affected area, making sure that the area is well saturated (fig. 4.4).

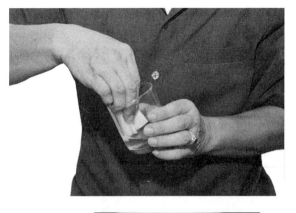

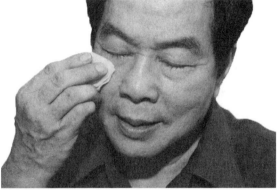

Fig. 4.4. External urine therapy

3. Discard the pad and saturate another clean pad with urine and reapply, lightly patting and soaking the affected area. Continue reapplying in this manner for 5–10 minutes or as many times as desired; the more the affected area is treated, the better.

4. Secure a clean soaked pad to the affected area with a gauze or cotton wrap and leave secured for several hours for additional healing. These urine packs are also incredibly effective for any type of insect sting, bite, or poison oak or ivy (see "urine packs and compresses" below).

5. Another method is to pour old or fresh urine into a clean, plastic spray bottle and spray the rash.

☢ *Skin Massages*

These massages have a tonifying, refreshing, relaxing effect and are said to allow for gradual absorption of urine nutrients through the skin. This practice is recommended especially when fasting for an acute condition, and people who use it swear by it. However, do not attempt these massages on extremely elderly or infirm individuals.

If you are using oral urine therapy, you should make it a point to add these skin massages of the face, neck, and feet.

1. Pour either old or fresh urine into a wide, shallow container and dip your hands into the liquid.
2. Shake off excess, then vigorously massage into a small area of skin anywhere on the body until hands and skin are dry.
3. Rewet hands and begin massaging another area until dry; repeat this step until all skin areas have been well massaged.
4. Rinse with warm water.

Make certain that you use normal urine for massages. If your own urine is dark, turbid, or abnormal looking, wait until you have taken urine internally over the course of two or three days, at which time the urine usually appears clear and can then be used for massages. Urine from a normal healthy person other than yourself may also be used for your external massage. If you are a heavy smoker, or are taking therapeutic or recreational drugs, you must begin urine therapy very gradually to avoid strong symptoms of detoxification. (See pages 111–12 for more information.)

☢ *Cosmetic Applications*

As the research studies show, urea replenishes the water content of the skin because it binds hydrogen and attracts moisture to the skin in a way that no mineral oil or glycerin-based lotions or creams can. You will be absolutely amazed at the softness and beauty of your skin after even one treatment with a urine massage. Old dead skin immediately flakes away, and your skin becomes wonderfully soft, rosy, and with time, even less wrinkled. Urine massages have also been reported to eliminate varicose veins and cysts.

1. For cosmetic use or moisturizing, pour a very small amount of normal fresh urine, or urine that has been stored for a day or two, into your hand and massage lightly into the skin until dry; then pour additional urine into your hand, massage it into another area of the skin until dry and so on.

2. Rinse well with warm water when completed, but wash without soap. Your skin is naturally slightly acidic, which gives it a natural protective coating. Because soaps are alkaline, they diminish the skin's acidity and thereby make it more vulnerable to moisture loss.

3. You can apply a moisturizer after the massage, but make sure that it is a simple, natural one that does not contain a lot of drying alcohol or other chemicals. You can also add a few drops of urine to your moisturizing cream each time you apply it.

◔ Eye and Nose Drops

You can use urine drops as both eye and nose drops, for relief of itchy or inflamed eyes, or for nasal congestion. In each case, make certain that you are using fresh, clear, normal urine only, and that it has normal acidity.

Urine Packs and Compresses

Urine packs and compresses are an invaluable tool for treating many external disorders, including bites and stings, tumors, and rashes. They have also been used successfully for arthritic and rheumatic pains.

❃ *Additional Healing for Skin Disorders*

Urine packs give added healing to skin disorders such as eczema, psoriasis, athlete's foot, ringworm, poison ivy and oak, and others.

1. Soak gauze bandages or cotton balls in fresh or old urine and place them over the affected areas.
2. Cover the urine pack with light plastic wrap and tape or tie it in place.
3. Try to keep the pack on as long as possible, especially with more severe conditions. Add additional urine to the pack with a medicine dropper every few hours to keep the pack wet.

❃ *Bites and Stings*

The pain and irritation of bee stings, mosquito bites, and other insect bites and stings are wonderfully relieved by this method.

❃ *Snakebite*

Urine packs should also be used immediately for poisonous snakebites. Follow emergency first aid instructions to rinse the wound and remove venom, if possible. Then apply fresh normal urine to the wound and secure a well-soaked urine pack over it. Keep pack wet until medical help can be obtained.

❃ *Growths and Tumors*

Urine compresses can be remarkably effective in reducing and eradicating a wide variety of internal and external tumors, cysts, and abnormal growths.

1. Compresses should be used in combination with internal urine therapy for treating any type of abnormal growth.
2. In preparing a compress, use a thick pad of clean white cotton material (like an old T-shirt), folded multiple times to increase its thickness.
3. Warm fresh or old urine by pouring it into a glass jar, then placing the jar in a container of hot water for a few minutes. When the urine is warm, soak the pad in it.
4. While lying down, place your wet compress over the affected area and cover with a clean folded towel. Keep the compress applied for as long as possible, reapplying warm urine as needed to keep the compress wet.

◎ Wounds, Burns, and Abrasions

As so many research and clinical studies have shown, urea is a tremendously effective antibacterial agent and an excellent healing treatment for wounds and burns of all types. Many people have applied urine compresses to burns and cuts with amazing results. The pain is quickly relieved and the burn or wound heals rapidly without scarring. Use fresh, normal urine for treating open wounds.

1. Saturate a thick gauze bandage or cotton pad with fresh urine, place it over the wound or burn and secure it with additional gauze; cover with plastic or soft towel to prevent leakage.
2. Reapply fresh urine with a clean medicine dropper directly onto the existing inside compress. Apply a fresh compress as often as possible.

Urine is also known to prevent scarring, so keep the urine pack applied as long or as often as possible until healing is complete.

Urine Therapy—Internal Use

Begin with Oral Drops

Start by taking only few drops each day in order to let your body adjust gradually.

Fill a clean medicine dropper from a fresh cup of morning, midstream urine, and place one or two drops under your tongue. This method lets you get used to the taste slowly and will still give you health benefits.

1. Start by taking 1–5 drops of morning urine on the first day.
2. The second day, take 5–10 drops in the morning.
3. Third day, take 5–10 drops in the morning, and the same amount in the evening before you go to bed.
4. Once you feel accustomed to the therapy, gradually increase the amount as needed, until you begin to see changes in your condition. As you use urine therapy, you will learn to adjust the amount you need by observing your reactions to it (fig. 4.5).

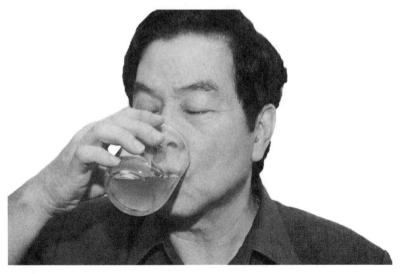

Fig. 4.5. Internal urine therapy

Do Not Boil or Dilute Urine

Research studies show that boiling urine destroys many of its medicinal properties, so when taking it internally, use it only in its fresh, natural form. Studies have also shown that diluting urine (or urea) decreases its antibacterial activity, so gradually increase your dosage rather than diluting it in juice or water to get accustomed to the taste.

Detoxification Symptoms

When you first begin urine therapy, you may initially experience detoxification symptoms such as headache, nausea, diarrhea, tiredness, or skin rashes. These are the body's natural responses to stored toxins being excreted and removed from the body, and they normally disappear within 24 to 36 hours. If you experience unpleasant symptoms with urine therapy, you can decrease the amount you are ingesting and continue with smaller doses. Or, you may avoid or lessen the severity of detoxification altogether by starting your therapy with a few oral drops. Homeopathic remedies and simple herbs are often of great help during detoxification to relieve headache, nausea, diarrhea, etc.

Monitor and Balance Your pH

It is extremely important to monitor your pH levels during urine therapy because if your urine is too alkaline, its antibacterial activity may decrease. On the other hand, if the urine is consistently or excessively acidic, urine therapy could create too much of an acid burden on your body.

It is always good to keep an eye on both your urine and saliva pH levels, because both should present a proper acid/alkaline balance. The ideal pH range of saliva is about 6.4–7.2, (below 6.4 is too acidic, above 7.2 is too alkaline). Saliva usually becomes more alkaline after eating and with a vegetarian diet. Urine pH should ideally vary from approximately 5.0 (acid in the morning) to 8.0 (alkaline at night) during each 24-hour period. If your urine or saliva pH levels are consistently out of range for a long period of time, it means that your body is not functioning correctly or that your diet is consistently too acidic or too alkaline.

Morning urine is generally more acidic than mid-day urine, and pH also changes in response to diet—in general, foods like meats, coffee, alcohol, milk, eggs, and beans make the body more acidic, while most fruits and vegetables have an alkalizing effect. Chronic over-acidity is called acidosis, and can be caused by such things as kidney, liver, or adrenal disorders, improper diet, starvation, anger, stress, fear, fever, or even excess vitamin C, aspirin, or niacin. Symptoms may include insomnia, water retention, migraine headaches, frequent sighing, abnormally low blood pressure, dry hard stools, alternating constipation and diarrhea, sensitivity of the teeth, difficulty swallowing, and recessed eyes.

Alkalosis (when the body is too alkaline) can be caused by such things as excessive use of antacids, a poor diet, excessive vomiting (bulimia), endocrine imbalances, high cholesterol, osteoarthritis, or diarrhea. Symptoms may include drowsiness, protruding eyes, creaking joints, sore muscles, bursitis, edema, night coughs, menstrual problems, allergies, night cramps, chronic indigestion, or asthma.

The first and easiest ways to correct pH are to increase relaxation, rest, fresh air, and exercise, while decreasing stress and adjusting your diet as recommended in chapter 1. If you have a severe chronic problem with acidosis, as is often the case with diabetics, use only a few drops of urine at a time, or substitute a homeopathic urine preparation.

You can easily monitor your pH at home with commercially available test strips that measure your acid/alkaline levels and show you their numerical values. Test your urine pH once or twice each day for a few days when using urine therapy for the first time, or when using it intensively. Do not ingest the same urine that you dip the pH strip into for testing. If you are taking only a small maintenance dose per day, test pH once every three to five days in order to determine whether dietary adjustments are needed. If you find that your urine pH is very acidic, add a pinch of baking soda to the urine you will be ingesting to reduce the acidity.

If You Are Pregnant, Do Not Use Urine Therapy without a Doctor's Supervision

Although pregnant women have been treated successfully with urine therapy for morning sickness or edema, the therapy should not be used during pregnancy without the supervision of a doctor familiar with the medical use of urine. While some doctors have obtained excellent results using urine therapy for morning sickness, there are reports of two spontaneous abortions that occurred after urine therapy treatments. It is possible that these miscarriages were caused by the natural release of toxins that occurs with urine therapy.

Urine Therapy and Fertility

On the other hand, if you're trying to get pregnant, you may already know that several successful fertility drugs such as Pergonal are made from urine extracts. Many women have reported that they feel urine therapy helped them to conceive. The best and safest method in this case is to use urine therapy for a certain time period (six months) before trying to conceive and to discontinue its use during the days that you are attempting to conceive. You can use urine diagnostic tests to determine when you are ovulating and when you have conceived, and you can gear your use of urine accordingly.

Urine Therapy and Drug Use

Traditionally, urine therapy has been discouraged for heavy smokers, drug users (including those on medications), and alcohol and coffee drinkers. However, new research shows that urine therapy can be beneficial under all of these conditions. Dr. William Hitt, an American doctor who owns urine therapy clinics in Mexico, has reported that he has treated 20,000 patients in a two-and-a-half-year period with urine therapy injections. These patients include those with cancer, asthma, and other diseases, and also patients with severe alcoholism, drug addictions, and smoking addictions. Dr. Hitt reports startling success with no side effects using urine injections for addictive disorders and also in combination with prescription drugs. The amount of drugs or contaminants passed into urine is so infinitesimal that they pose no threat and, in fact, appear to act as vaccine-type agents that improve or cure these types of disorders. This view is also supported by the book *Urinalysis in Clinical Laboratory Practice* (Alfred H. Free and Helen Free. Cleveland: CRC Press; 1977), in which the authors state that even in cases of severe mercury poisoning, the amount of actual mercury passed into the urine is infinitesimal.

When contaminants like drugs and alcohol are present in the body, begin urine therapy with 1–5 drops orally per day for 3–5 days, in order to avoid heavy detoxification symptoms. Increase the dosage by one or two drops each day, according to how well you're tolerating the therapy, then gradually increase the amount as needed to obtain results for your individual condition.

Improve Your Diet and Limit Meat when Using Urine Therapy

In general, your diet should consist of balanced amounts of whole grains, fresh vegetables, and small amounts of lean meats and fish. If you are ingesting large amounts of refined foods, sugar, soda, and coffee you will not get the full benefits of urine therapy and, depending on how poor your diet is, you may experience unpleasant symptoms, such as headache or nausea, as your body regulates and expels undesirable elements. If you are only using a few oral drops of urine or ingesting one or two ounces once a day, your meat intake can remain normal as long as "normal" for you is moderate.

As studies on urea and the kidney have shown, urea helps your body break down proteins more efficiently, which may mean that when using urine therapy, you can get the benefits of increased protein intake even though you are eating less meat and other sources of protein. This information will probably also be of value to vegetarians who rely on much less concentrated protein sources in their foods than meat eaters. Decrease or eliminate meat in your diet while ingesting large amounts of urine or preparing for a fast, as combining intensive urine therapy and high meat intake may lead to excess acid levels in the body.

Homeopathic Urine

Homeopathic urine is a greatly diluted preparation that allows you to receive many of the benefits of oral urine therapy with fewer potential side effects and greater ease of administration. It also allows you to use urine collected at the beginning or height of acute symptoms of illness—particularly symptoms of infection and allergy—without fear of spoilage. Many researchers emphasize this urine collected during illness as particularly potent, because it contains the greatest amount of antibodies and immune-defense agents that the body is using to fight the illness. A homeopathic preparation preserves this potent first-stage-illness urine and can then be used throughout the duration of it. Homeopathic urine is also excellent for children, and for those with extreme sensitivity or toxicity who feel they are reacting too strongly to fresh urine therapy.

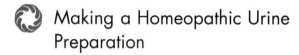 ## Making a Homeopathic Urine Preparation

You can make a homeopathic preparation of urine as follows:

1. Put 5 ml (0.169 ounces) of distilled water in a clean, dry bottle or jar with a close-fitting lid. Add 1 drop of fresh urine, then cap the bottle and shake vigorously 50 times.

2. Put one drop of this solution into another clean, dry jar. To this 1
drop of solution, add another 5 ml of distilled water. Shake vigorously 50 times.
3. Take 1 drop of this new solution and add it to 5 ml of 80- to
90-proof vodka.

To use this homeopathic preparation, place 3 drops under the
tongue each hour, until there is either an obvious improvement or
a temporary flare-up of the symptoms. As the patient improves, the
time between treatments can be lengthened. Treatment should be
stopped after three days, allowing the immune system to take over.
Repeated treatment is necessary only if the patient's progress becomes
static or if a relapse of the condition occurs.

Urine Therapy for Children

Several research studies deal specifically with the treatment of children with urine therapy. The easiest way to administer it is with oral
drops of the child's own fresh urine. For treatment of acute colds, flu,
or other viral infections like measles, mumps, chicken pox, and so
forth, small frequent oral doses of 1–10 drops during illness have been
shown to be very effective. For allergies, several drops of fresh urine
should be given orally before and after meals containing allergenic
foods, or when allergic symptoms are present.

As with adults, symptoms of illness may temporarily increase in
children immediately following the first few doses of urine therapy,
but, in all cases, these symptoms dissipated within 24–48 hours. For
ear infections, fresh, warm urine drops in the affected ear can give
excellent and often instantaneous results. Repeat as needed.
Another very effective method is to prepare a homeopathic dilution of
the child's urine for use throughout the illness or allergy attack. See
the section "Homeopathic Urine" on page 113 for more details about
this method.

Urine Therapy Maintenance Dose

For people who use urine therapy regularly, a daily maintenance dose is usually considered to be one to two ounces of morning midstream urine, but this dose may also be as little as 5–10 drops per day, or every other day, depending on your individual condition and needs. Many lifetime users of urine therapy (including the former prime minister of India) have commented that regular use of urine therapy noticeably assists in maintaining energy levels, reducing aging, and in preventing illness.

Severe, Acute, and Chronic Illnesses

If you are suffering from an acute illness like an infection, the traditional treatment is to fast completely or to eat only light meals (such as homemade, unseasoned vegetable broth) while ingesting frequent doses of urine for at least one day, or until you feel that your improvement is complete and stable. I have found, as have many others, that eating heavily too soon after recovering from a viral or bacterial infection may produce a relapse, so make sure that you're feeling stable before starting to eat normally again. Always break your fast by slowly reintroducing light foods, homemade fresh vegetable soups, then crackers, grains, and so forth.

For those with chronic or severe illnesses like cancer, some urine therapy users strongly recommend ingesting as much urine as you pass, or as much as possible during the day for several days, although much smaller doses have also been reported to be effective. If you are ingesting large amounts of urine, it may be a good idea to fast or sharply decrease your solid food intake during this time; this will reduce the burden on your kidneys and allow your body to use more energy for healing, rather than digestion. Short urine and water fasts of 1–3 days, as described in more detail on pages 118–19, can be very effective therapy. However, it would be extremely unadvisable for most people to undertake any kind of prolonged urine fast.

If you do not want to fast, but feel that you need to ingest larger amounts of urine, eat small, simple meals—preferably, fresh home-made unseasoned vegetable soups. If you feel you need a grain, use plain millet, rice, or another whole grain, and salt-free crackers. Long-standing, difficult conditions may naturally require a longer period of treatment, during which you are likely to vary your food and urine intake from time to time. What I discovered in my own treatment was that I needed to ingest a large amount of urine initially—about 2 ounces 4–5 times/day—every day for about two weeks, at which point I switched to small frequent doses of 1–2 ounces three to four times a day. After another two weeks I tapered off to 1–2 ounces twice a day, then every other day, and so forth. My maintenance dose is 5–10 drops per day. This was my approach, but you may find that your individual requirements are more or less than these amounts.

Rest, Rest, Rest

Assiduous urine therapy can give you such renewed vigor and energy that it's easy to become overconfident and overdo life. Although over-doing it may not be a huge problem for normal people, exhaustion is a life-long threat for people recovering from major illnesses. Once you have healed a serious illness and achieved improved health, continue the practice of a daily maintenance dose of urine therapy and a good diet, and never allow yourself to become consistently exhausted or overtired. Consistent, proper rest is much more crucial to health than most people realize.

There are many instances in which people completely cure themselves of even "incurable" diseases through urine therapy and natural healing and remain well for a number of years, only to completely undo all the good they have accomplished by overconfidently pushing themselves to extremes in their work or recreation. One of the saddest examples of this was the case of a young, bright, determined AIDS patient who had completely cured himself of all visible and clinical evidence of the disease, but subsequently consistently and relentlessly overworked himself at his demanding corporate job. Eventually, he fell ill, relapsed, and was unable to recover.

However, in another case, a person who had recovered from a serious illness experienced a relapse from overexertion, but recovered again with complete rest and intense urine therapy. Why put yourself through another ordeal and risk the chance of seriously undermining your body's hard-earned repair work? Protect your newfound health and your natural immune defenses with lots of rest, fresh air, moderate exercise, and minimized stress.

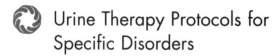 Urine Therapy Protocols for Specific Disorders

Allergies

Begin with one or two oral drops, and then gradually increase the amount until you can no longer sense the urine taste or temperature. If you know what your allergies are, take the drops before eating a food that you are allergic to. If you do not know what you are allergic to, take several drops of fresh urine immediately upon the appearance of symptoms, and repeat this method each time the symptoms recur. Homeopathic urine preparations as described above are also excellent for allergies, as you can preserve the urine collected at the height of allergy symptoms for long-term treatment of the allergy.

Food Poisoning

Several research studies show that urea is a proven antibacterial agent, even containing antibodies to food contaminants such as salmonella bacteria in infected individuals. Begin by taking 1–5 drops. Increase dosage as tolerated.

Kidney Disorders

If you have a current or past kidney infection, limit the initial amount of oral urine you take to small doses such as 1–5 drops once or twice a day. Decrease or eliminate the consumption of meat and acid-forming foods before beginning the therapy. Also, check your acidity levels with pH strips as described above, and begin urine therapy when your acid levels have normalized or decreased substantially.

Fasting on Urine

Fasting on urine is an excellent therapy that can produce extraordinary results, especially for intractable diseases and tough chronic conditions, but always work into a fast slowly. Pushing your body too quickly can produce severe detoxifying symptoms such as headaches, fever, nausea, depression, or fatigue that you can lessen or avoid by simply adjusting to the therapy gradually with a few oral drops each day.

Short periods of fasting (1–3 days) can be an extremely effective method for cleansing and healing the body; long fasts should always be undertaken with caution and supervision. Be sure to eliminate all meat intake for at least three days before you begin fasting.

1. Begin taking oral drops of urine for two to three weeks, while continuing to eat normally.
2. Increase your dosage to 1–3 ounces during the next two or three weeks.
3. Begin fasting the following week. During the fast, ingest as much urine as you pass during the day until it becomes completely clear; stop ingesting it for a few hours and then resume.
4. Decrease or stop your intake at night and begin again when you awaken in the morning.

Alternate urine intake with small sips of cool water or ice chips if desired. Drink as much water as you feel thirsty for, and stay well hydrated at all times, but do not force-drink large quantities of water, as research shows this can dilute the urine and decrease its antibacterial action. Force-drinking water in combination with urine ingestion may also stress the kidneys.

Combine urine fasting with urine skin massages, particularly on the face, neck, and feet. This gives extra nourishment to the body during fasting and eliminates possible headaches and nausea. The rubs are also refreshing and make the skin clear and soft. When breaking your fast, start by eating a simple homemade fresh vegetable soup broth made of fresh kale, carrots, fresh green leeks, scallion tops, and a little fresh ginger. Do not add salt or seasonings. Eat only the broth for a day or two, the broth and vegetable the next day, and begin gradually adding in more vegetables and carbohydrates such as rice and millet over the next few days.

Dos of Oral Urine Therapy

- Start with small amounts and work up to larger amounts gradually.
- Use only fresh urine.
- Test your pH to make certain that you are not overly acidic before taking urine internally, and continue to monitor your pH periodically during your course of therapy.

Don'ts of Oral Urine Therapy

- Don't rush into the therapy with large amounts.
- Don't combine urine therapy with a starvation diet (or fasting) unless you have been using the therapy for at least two months.
- Don't continue to work while fasting on urine therapy. If you are ingesting large amounts of urine and fasting, you must rest and relax in order to avoid possibly stressing the kidneys.
- Don't ingest large amounts of urine while eating a consistently acidic diet.

A Testimonial to Urine Therapy

This following account is presented not as a prescription but as a simple telling of one family's experiences with urine therapy.

Twelve years ago I was bitten by a dog. I was riding my bicycle with our two-year-old son on my shoulders. The dog rushed me from the side, bit into the ankle and held on twisting and pulling. His handler immediately began to pull the guard dog off me as I struggled to not have my son fall. Finally the dog was off and I was able to bike about 200 meters to our home. Our son fell into my wife's arms and I flopped on the ground writhing in pain.

The gash from the bite was ugly and deep. Our six-year-old ran up to me and right away peed directly into the wound. My wife and the other children grabbed a clean bucket and everyone took turns urinating into it. Other people arrived and told us I should go to the hospital without delay. We were in the tropics and bites can be dangerous and fatal. Instead, I sat with the injured ankle in a bucket full of the family's fresh urine. We were a family of six at the time and so it was rather easy to keep the fresh urine coming. I also drank my own urine several times a day. We had used urine with good results on insect bites, scratches, and cuts. Once we were able to get the children through a feverish sickness resulting from coral cuts through the applications of urine compresses. Kids do not seem to need to drink great amounts of their urine to achieve relief and rebound back into robust health.

This dog bite was pretty scary but the reaction of my body to the urine therapy was very strong and positive. I had a raging and raving fever that night and my wife made use of refrigerated urine that had been boiled down to an oily, thick liquid. She massaged it into my skin over the whole body. She used a cool urine compress on my forehead. I remember that sensation of blessed coolness and my wife's strong, caring massage. I spent the next day sitting quietly, always with that bucket being emptied and refilled by the family. I continued to drink my urine output. The following day I wrapped a urine-soaked bandana around the wounded but healing ankle. I was feeling stronger by the hour and the gash itself appeared to be mending. I went out to do my work always with a urine-soaked gauze and bandana. In fact, after four days I was hiking in the jungle with the family and friends.

So that is the story of dog bites man, children pee into wound, family urine bucket, and using urine to overcome a dangerous injury.

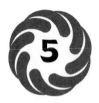

Maintenance and Prevention

Many people are occasionally inspired to undertake a fast or a cleanse or a new healthy diet, but the fact is that these measures can only take you so far; the more profound healing experiences come with the smaller alterations of daily habits. This notion may seem daunting, but the process of changing for the better is one that is properly accomplished over time, step by step, as you gradually integrate new ways of eating, cleansing, and thinking. As your daily behaviors become a result of choice rather than habit, you are on your way to developing effective strategies of maintenance and prevention.

The best place to begin is with your diet. Try to keep your food intake 80 percent alkaline-forming foods. This will assist your body greatly in its daily detoxification efforts. In addition, follow the time-tested guidelines below. Good luck!

Living Guidelines for Maintenance and Prevention

- Eat on an empty stomach.
- Drink only water between meals (okay to add lemon juice and cayenne pepper).
- Never eat after 6:00 p.m. (herb teas are okay).

- Eat 2–3 small meals per day, between 10 a.m. and 6 p.m.
- Don't eat big meals.
- Never eat candy, cakes, or other junk food.
- Never drink soda pop, coffee, or caffeinated tea.
- Never eat breads, sweetened cereals, or other white flour products.
- Eat raw salads containing 4 or 5 of the following: celery, onion, lemon, peppers, romaine, tomato, cabbage.
- Eat steamed green vegetables including broccoli, kale, cabbage, beet tops, spinach, chard.
- Eat steamed tubers including yams, beets, carrots, and rutabagas (okay to add coconut oil or olive oil).
- Do not eat meat (chicken or fish) at the same meal as starches or tubers.
- Eat legume soups made from beans or lentils and garlic, sea salt, pepper, and olive oil.
- Eat whole grain cereals like rye, rice, or oats (Okay to add soaked dried fruits, seeds, nuts, cinnamon, or ginger).
- Fast on Mondays (water only).
- Don't use tobacco in any form, or chew gum.
- Never eat lying down; always sit up straight.
- Do not eat when you're tired or upset, only when you're at peace.

THE FOURTEEN-DAY CLEANSE FOR THE NINE OPENINGS

In addition to following the dietary guidelines suggested above, it is a good idea to properly cleanse your body's nine openings every six months. To do so, you should set aside two weeks twice a year for the following practices.

Cleansing Drinks and Supplements: The Cellular Cleanse

Eat nothing for 14 days. During this time, drink the following 2 drinks in succession, 5 times per day.

> **1st Drink:** Place the juice from one lime, 8 ounces of pure water, 1 tablespoon of bentonite, and 1 teaspoon of psyllium into a jar. Shake for 15 seconds, and drink quickly.
>
> **2nd Drink:** 10 ounces pure water, 1 tablespoon apple cider vinegar, 1 teaspoon maple syrup. Place all ingredients in a jar, shake for 15 seconds, and drink quickly.

On the days indicated in the chart below, take the recommended supplements 4 times per day, 1.5 hours after your drinks.

SUPPLEMENT SCHEDULE (4 times per day)

	Day 1	Day 2	Days 3, 7 & 14
Chlorophyll gel tablets	12	18	24
Vitamin C tablets	200 mg	200 mg	800 mg
Pancreatin tablets	6	6	6
Beet tablets	2	2	2
Dulse tablets	1	1	1
Enzymatic tablets	2	2	2
Niacin tablets	50 mg	100 mg	200 mg
Wheat germ oil tablets	1	1	1

Other Cleansing Practices

The following cleanses for the nine openings should be done during the same two weeks as the cellular cleanse described above.

> **Colonics:** One colonic every other day for two weeks, either self-administered or with a colon therapist. Include the following implants: coffee and garlic; garlic and Epsom salts; acidophilus (final day)
>
> **Ear Candling:** Use 2 candles per ear with an assistant during cleanse.
>
> **Mouth Flush:** At separate times, gargle hydrogen peroxide, baking soda, and olive oil.
>
> **Nasal Flush:** Use Real Salt in warm water to douche nasal cavities.
>
> **Eye Flush:** Use lemon juice or apple cider vinegar in warm water to douche eyes.
>
> **Solar Bathing:** Expose body to open air and sun.
>
> **Dry Skin Brushing:** Brush before morning bath and before bed at night.

Liver/Gallbladder Flush

Do flush the day before last colonic.

> **Ingredients:** Epsom salts, olive oil, squeezed grapefruit, ornithine
>
> **Preparation:** Drink 32 ounces of apple juice the day before flush.
>
> **2:00 p.m.** Do not eat or drink after 2:00 p.m. Mix 4 tablespoons Epsom salts in 3 cups water for 4 servings (¾ cup each). Set jar in refrigerator.
>
> **6:00 p.m.** Drink 1st Epsom salts serving (¾ cup).
>
> **8:00 p.m.** Drink 2nd Epsom salts serving (¾ cup).

9:45 p.m. Mix ½ cup olive oil and ¾ cup fresh-squeezed grapefruit juice in a pint jar.

10:00 p.m. Shake olive oil/grapefruit mix and drink with a straw. Take 8 capsules of L-Ornithine with this drink. Lie down immediately, and keep still for 20 min. Go to sleep right away.

6:00 a.m. Drink 3rd Epsom salts serving (¾ cup). Go back to bed.

8:00 a.m. Drink 4th Epsom salts serving (¾ cup). You may go back to bed.

10:00 a.m. You may eat. Expect diarrhea, passing tan and green gallstones.

11:00 a.m. Take final colonic with acidophilus implant.

Ending the Six-Month Cleanse

Breaking Cleanse: Add parsley and garlic to asparagus.

Kidney Flush: Steam 5 bunches of asparagus and eat it as 3 separate meals over the course of 1.5 days. Also drink 1 quart of cranberry juice for 2 days.

Conclusion

As energy continues to flow through the cleanses and you gain more and more confidence in letting go, a strange thing happens. You learn that the universe is moving through you all the time, and if you let it, your life becomes effortless. This really is the path of the Tao—the effortless path. Although the life force that moves through everything is very strong, we resist its flow through bad eating habits or by hanging onto cultural conditioning instead of letting go. When you hang on to old thoughts or habits, you block this marvelous flow. But when you let go, the flow will eventually pick you up and take you where you are supposed to go. The flow knows where it is going, so you don't really need to. You will experience it spontaneously: that really is the flow of the universe, the flow of our own energy vibrating.

This is the effortless path. You open yourself up to it when you are detached from all the other connections in life. We really are as free as birds, we just complicate things by going out and desiring things that are not really necessary for us in our lives. This leads to pain and suffering, because you are swimming against the river. So the nine-openings cleanse every six months will clean out your river on a regular basis to maintain your connection with the Tao.

We are the Creator of what we are and we can manifest whatever we want. This is the message of the Tao. Through this system of cleansing you can prepare yourself to become an Immortal and break the karmic wheel in one sojourn, or live a long healthy life following your bliss.

Life is simple and complete once you have the concept of what you are doing. The concept creates the desire to manifest what you want. This is the whole process of becoming, from the initial manifestation of the physical realm to every thought we have: concept, desire, and manifestation. In these pages, we have given you the concept of cleansing your nine openings, which will give you the desire to do it.

It is the same process for all of us: just think it and you will become it. So become your own reality with the help of the knowledge and wisdom in this book.

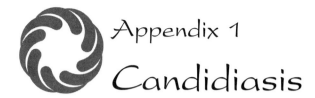

Appendix 1
Candidiasis

Candidiasis has become a "hot" topic over the past few years among health-conscious individuals in the United States. It is a condition that results from the overgrowth of yeast (a type of fungus), most commonly the one called *Candida albicans*. Candida cells are part of the normal flora of our bodies found in the mouth, vagina, intestines, and other organs, but if they multiply out of proportion to other kinds of cells, they can cause a number of health problems including digestive disorders, fatigue, and vaginal yeast infections. Whether candidiasis is to be considered a disease or a syndrome is still controversial in conventional medicine, but the general public has accepted it as a valid disease, apart from lab tests or theoretical constructs. Some practitioners even claim that "everybody" has it.

Traditional Chinese medicine recognizes the development and proliferation of candida as a condition related primarily to the spleen. The spleen is responsible for taking the food and fluids that we ingest and processing them into the chi and blood that are the true "fuel" of our bodies. When the spleen is functioning well, chi and blood are in balance, intestinal flora are in balance, there is no excess fluid or phlegm in the system, food is properly digested and distributed, and the immune system is nourished.

However, when spleen energy is weakened by poor diet, medications, or other factors, its ability to transform food is diminished. Unable to properly absorb and utilize nutrients from the foods we eat, the spleen then can't produce healthy amounts of chi and blood. If treated appropriately at this stage—with a re-balancing of the spleen and stomach energies—the problem will resolve with no yeast-related symptoms. But candidiasis is not a well-defined disease pattern. It is difficult to diagnose at the early stages, and many people are completely unaware that they are developing a severe problem when they experience symptoms such as digestive disorders, irregular bowel movements, diarrhea, constipation, and/or fatigue. In the absence of treatment, or with improper treatment, the disorder will then spread from the spleen and the Spleen meridian to other organs and meridians, resulting in symptoms such as fatigue, headaches, thrush, cheesy vaginal discharge, genital itching, or vaginitis. At this stage, the condition will be diagnosed as a systemic yeast infection.

Chinese Medicine Two-Step Treatment Plan for Candidiasis

Step 1. A thorough cleansing is the first step in dealing with candidiasis. When our systems are full of the waste, phlegm, and toxins that contribute to yeast overgrowth, clearing them out is necessary. "The constitutional energy is endangered when an internalized evil is there," says the *Yellow Emperor's Classic of Internal Medicine.* Many people try to clear out their yeast overgrowth with dietary changes, but diet management alone is not generally enough to clear the system entirely of candida; if it does work, it will take a very long time.

However, combining proper diet with Chinese herbs and acupuncture can achieve this goal much faster. With herbal cleansing therapy, the goal is to clear the system of dampness, phlegm, and heat. These are seen as the causative factors of candidiasis. The herbs are not intended to mechanically clear out the large intestine; rather, they promote the clearing-out of the pathological factors of phlegm and heat toxins.

Damp Heat Clearing Formula

Boil the following ingredients together for 20 minutes, then steep for three hours. Drink 2–3 times per day on an empty stomach. Continue for 1–2 weeks then stop.

Gentian Formula (Long Dan Xie Gan Tang)

Gentian (Long Dan Cao)—2 parts
Bupleurum (Chai Hu)—2 parts
Alisma (Ze Xie)—2 parts
Scullcap (Huang Qin)—1 part
Gardenia (Zhi Zi)—1 part
Akebia (Mu Tong)—1 part
Plaintain (Che Qian Cao)—1 part
Rehmannia (Di Huang)—1 part
Angelica (Dang Gui)—1 part
Licorice (Gan Cao)—1 part

To enhance the effectiveness of this damp heat formula, some commonly used acupuncture/acupressure points for this cleansing process include LV3, LV2, ST40, UB57, and LI4.

Step 2. Tonifying: After the waste, toxins, and phlegm have been cleared out of our systems, we then need to tonify our bodies, repairing the damage and restoring the balance so the pathological factor(s) do not return. "If sufficient vital energy exists, a pathological factor cannot attack us," explains the *Yellow Emperor's Classic of Internal Medicine*. This is a very important step for preventing recurrence of a yeast infection. Commonly used tonifying herbs include astragalus (huang qi), codonopsis (dang shen), atractylodes (bai zhu), and dioscorea (shan yao). The GI Strength Formula (Xian Sha Liu Jun Zi Tang) described below is a popular formula for tonification, especially of the Middle Heater.

⊙ GI Strength Formula (Xian Sha Liu Jun Zi Tang)

Boil the following ingredients together for 20 minutes, then steep for 3 hours. Drink over a period of a week.

Fresh ginger (Sheng Jiang)—2 parts
Atractylodes (Bai Zhu)—2 parts
Poria (Fu Ling)—2 parts
Ginseng (Ren Shen)—1 part
Pinella (Ban Xia)—1 part
Licorice (Gan Cao)—1 part
Tangerine Peel (Chen Pi)—1 part
Amomum (Sha Ren)—1 part
Saussurea (Mu Xiang)—1part

To enhance the effectiveness of the tonifying formula, some commonly used tonifying acupuncture/acupressure points include ST36, SP9, SP6, LI10, LV8, CV6, and CV4.

⊙ Recommendations for Your Diet

People who are familiar with a yeast-free diet stay away from bread, cheese, mushrooms, vinegar, soy sauce, barbecue sauce, black fungus, and white fungus. But there are other yeast-based foods such as crackers, pretzels, dry cereal, miso, tempeh, canned vegetables, pickled vegetables, beer, root beer, and other fermented beverages that are often overlooked by those with yeast infections.

Grains, noodles, nonyeast bread, and white rice are recommended because they are easy to digest. Although brown rice and wild rice have more nutrients than white rice, they take more energy to digest, and it is better for spleen-chi-deficient people not to eat them often. Certain vegetables are extremely therapeutic for those with yeast infections, such as daikon radish, which can help cleanse your system and is known as a "phlegm cleanser." The family of yellow-colored foods such as yam, winter squash, and pumpkins are strongly recommended from the viewpoint of traditional Chinese medicine, as they tonify and strengthen the spleen and spleen meridian. Yeast-based medications such as penicillin, mycin, chloromycetin, and tetracyclines should be avoided, as well as yeast-based vitamin B supplements.

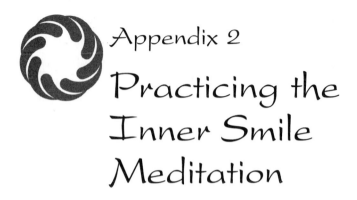

Appendix 2

Practicing the Inner Smile Meditation

The Inner Smile meditation is the most basic practice of the Universal Tao. It is a powerful relaxation and self-healing technique that uses the energy of happiness and love as a language to communicate with the internal organs of the body. A genuine smile transmits loving energy that has the power to calm, balance, and heal.

When you smile inwardly to the organs and glands your whole body feels loved and appreciated. The Inner Smile begins at the eyes and mid-eyebrow point. The eyes are connected to the autonomic nervous system, which in turn is connected to all the muscles, organs, and glands. As one of the first parts of the body to receive signals, the eyes cause the organs and glands to accelerate activity at times of stress or danger and to slow down when a crisis has passed. When the eyes relax, they activate the parasympathetic nervous system and cause the rest of the body to relax.

As you activate the loving energy, you will feel the energy of the Inner Smile flow down the entire length of the body like a waterfall. This is a very powerful and effective tool to counteract stress and tension.

There are three vital aspects to each phase of the Inner Smile. First, direct the awareness to a specific part of the body. Second, smile to that part of the body; send it a genuine feeling of love, gratitude, and appreciation for its role in keeping the body running smoothly and in good health. Third, feel that part of the body relax and smile back to you.

 ## The Inner Smile Practice

1. Stand in Wu Chi stance or sit on the edge of a chair with the hands comfortably clasped together and resting on the lap. Keep the eyes closed and breathe normally. Follow the breathing until it becomes smooth, quiet, deep, even, calm, and soft.

2. Relax the forehead. Imagine yourself in one of your favorite beautiful places in the world. Recall the sights, sounds, and sensations of that place until they are vividly in your mind's eye. Then imagine suddenly meeting someone you love. Picture him or her smiling lovingly and radiantly at you. Feel yourself basking in the warmth of that smile like sunshine, drawing it into your eyes. Feel the eyes relaxing and responding with a smile of their own.

3. Picture the healing chi of nature—the fresh energy of waterfalls, mountains, and oceans—as a golden cloud of benevolent loving energy in front of you. We call this the Higher Human Plane energy of the atmosphere, the blended chi of heaven and earth, or the Cosmic Particle force. Direct the smiling energy in the eyes to this Cosmic Particle energy around you, drawing it into the mid-eyebrow point. Feel the brow relaxing and widening. Spiral the energy into the mid-eyebrow point; feel it amplifying the power of your smile.

4. Let the smiling awareness flow down over the cheeks, down through the jaw muscles and tongue, and down through the neck and throat, soothing and relaxing as it goes.

5. Smile down to the thymus gland and the heart. Feel them open like flowers in the morning with love, joy, and happiness bubbling out of them.

6. Smile down to the rest of the solid organs: lungs, liver, pancreas,

spleen, kidneys, sexual organs, and reproductive system. Thank each of them for their work in keeping you vibrant and healthy. This completes the first line of the Inner Smile.

7. Return your awareness to your eyes and recharge the energy of your smile. Then draw in more of the golden light of the Cosmic Particle force.

8. Roll the tongue around the mouth until you have gathered some saliva. Smile to the saliva and draw the smiling energy and the golden light into the saliva, transforming it into a healing nectar.

9. Swallow the saliva in two or three strong gulps. Follow it with awareness down the esophagus, smiling as it goes, feeling the healing nectar soothing and refreshing the esophagus. Continue smiling through the rest of the digestive tract: the stomach, small intestine, gallbladder, large intestine, rectum, anus, bladder, and urethra. Thank these organs for their work in giving you energy through ingestion, digestion, absorption, and elimination. This completes the second or middle line of the Inner Smile.

10. Return your awareness to your eyes and recharge your smile. Then once again connect with the golden light of the Cosmic Particle force.

11. Now smile to the brain, to the left and right hemispheres, and to the pituitary, thalamus, and pineal glands. Then smile down through the spinal column vertebra by vertebra, thanking each vertebra for its work in protecting the spinal cord and supporting the skeletal structure. This completes the third or back line of the Inner Smile.

12. Return your awareness to your eyes once again and recharge your smiling energy.

13. Smile down through the whole body, particularly to any place that feels tired, sore, painful, weak, empty, or tense. Shower these parts with the healing nectar of your smiling awareness.

14. Finally, smile to the navel and collect the energy there.

15. Starting in the center of the navel, begin spiraling the energy outward. Men should spiral the energy in a clockwise direc-

tion, making thirty-six revolutions; women spiral the energy in a counterclockwise direction, also making thirty-six revolutions. Take care not to make the outer ring of the spiral any larger than a grapefruit; circling above the diaphragm causes too much energy to flow into the heart and overstimulates the emotions, whereas circling below the pubic bone sends too much energy into the reproductive system, where it may be lost through ejaculation or menses. After completing the first set of revolutions, spiral inward in the opposite direction twenty-four times, ending at the center of the navel.

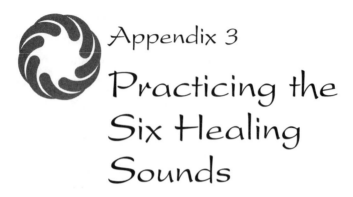

Appendix 3

Practicing the Six Healing Sounds

The Six Healing Sounds will help you sense the distinctive frequencies and colors generated by each organ. Practice the healing sounds until you can easily relate the sound to the organ and sense the qualities of that organ.

THE SIX HEALING SOUNDS INITIATE HEALING

Everyone has heard stories about gifted beings who possess special healing powers. People seek out great healers. How much time can a great healer spend with you—one hour a week or one hour every day? What about the rest of the week or the rest of the day? One hour a day means one hour out of twenty-four. One hour a week means one hour out of one hundred and sixty-eight. This is why it is important for each person to learn how to clear his or her own negative energy and how to transform it into good energy. Regular practice of self-maintenance and self-healing enhances ongoing healing. The Six Healing Sounds are an easy practice to initiate healing. The sounds are very simple but very powerful.

How to Make the Six Healing Sounds

The Lungs' Sound

Associated Organ: Large intestine
Element: Metal
Season: Autumn (dryness)
Color: White
Negative Emotions: Grief, sadness, depression, sorrow
Positive Emotions: Courage, righteousness, justice, detachment
Sound: Sss-s-s-s-s-s (tongue behind teeth)
Parts of the Body: Chest, inner arms, thumbs
Sense/Body Substance: Smell, nose, mucus, skin

1. Position: Sit with your back straight and the backs of your hand resting on your thighs. Smile down to your lungs. Take a deep breath and raise your arms out in front of you. When the hands are at eye level, begin to rotate the palms, bringing them above your head until they are palm up, pushing outward. Point the fingers toward those of the opposite hand. Keep the elbows rounded out to the side. Do not straighten your arms.

2. Sound: Close your jaw so that your teeth gently meet, and part your lips slightly. Inhale as you look up, eyes wide open, and push your palms upward and out as you slowly exhale through your teeth and make the sound "sss-s-s-s-s-s." At first you can produce the lungs' sound aloud, but eventually you should practice subvocally (vocalizing so softly that only you can hear the sound). Picture and feel excess heat, sick energy, sadness, sorrow, depression, and grief expelled as the pleura (the sacs surrounding the lungs) compress. Exhale slowly and fully.

3. Rest and concentrate: Resting is very important because during rest you can communicate with your inner self and your internal system. When you have exhaled completely, rotate the palms down as you slowly lower your shoulders, and return your hands to your lap, palms up. Close your eyes and be aware of your lungs. Smile into them and imagine that you are still making the lungs' sound. Breathe normally and picture your lungs growing with a bright white color. This will strengthen your lungs and draw down the universal energy associated with them. With each breath, try to feel the exchange of cool, fresh energy as it replaces excessively hot energy.

Repeat 6, 9, 12, or 24 times. Practice more often to alleviate sadness, depression, colds, flu, toothache, asthma, or emphysema.

☻ The Kidneys' Sound

Associated Organ: Urinary Bladder
Element: Water
Season: Winter
Color: Black or dark blue
Negative Emotions: Fear, shock
Positive Emotions: Gentleness, alertness, stillness, gratitude
Sound: Choo-oo-oo-oo (as when blowing out a candle with the lips forming an "O")
Parts of the Body: Side of foot, inner legs, chest
Sense/Body Substance: Hearing, ears, bones

1. Position: Bring your legs together, ankles and knees touching. Be aware of your kidneys and smile into them. Take a deep breath, lean forward, and clasp the fingers of both hands together around your knees. Pull your arms straight from your lower back while bending your torso forward. (This allows your back to protrude in the area of the kidneys.) Simultaneously tilt your head upward as you look straight ahead and maintain the pull on your arms from the lower back. Feel your spine pull.

2. Sound: Round your lips and slightly exhale the sound "choo-oo-oo-oo" as if you were blowing out a candle. Simultaneously contract your abdomen, pulling it in toward your kidneys. Imagine the excess heat, fear, and wet, sick energies squeezed out from the fascia surrounding the kidneys.

3. Rest and concentrate: After you have fully exhaled, sit erect, separate your legs, and place your hands on your thighs, palms up. Close your eyes, breathe into the kidneys, and be aware of them. Picture the bright color blue in the kidneys. Smile into them, imagining that you are still making the kidneys' sound. Repeat the above steps 3, 6, 12, or 24 times. Practice more often to alleviate fear, fatigue, dizziness, ringing in the ears, or back pain.

◐ The Liver's Sound

Associated Organ: Gallbladder
Element: Wood
Season: Spring
Color: Green
Negative Emotions: Anger, aggression
Positive Emotions: Kindness, generosity, forgiveness, self-expansion, identity
Sound: Sh-h-h-h-h-h-h (tongue near palate)
Parts of the Body: Inner legs, groin, diaphragm, ribs
Sense/Body Substance: Sight, eyes, tears

1. Position: Sit comfortably and straight. Be aware of the liver and smile into it. When you feel you are in touch with the liver, extend your arms out to your sides, palms up. Take a deep breath as you slowly raise your arms up and over your head from the sides, following this action with your eyes. Interlace your fingers and turn your joined hands over to face the ceiling, palms up. Push out at the heel of your palms and stretch your arms out from the shoulders. Bend slightly to the left, exerting a gentle pull on the liver.

2. Sound: Open your eyes wide, because they are the openings of the liver. Slowly exhale the sound "sh-h-h-h-h-h-h" subvocally.

Envision expelling excess heat and anger from the liver as the fasciae around it compress.

3. Rest and concentrate: When you have fully exhaled, separate your hands, turn the palms down, and slowly bring your arms down to your sides, leading with the heels of your hands. Breathe into the liver slowly and imagine a bright green color and quality of kindness entering the liver. Bring your hands to rest on your thighs, palms up. Smile down into the liver. Close your eyes, breathe into the liver, and imagine you are still making the liver's sound. Repeat 3, 6, 12, or 24 times. Practice more often to alleviate anger, soothe red or watery eyes, remove a sour or bitter taste, and detoxify the liver.

The Heart's Sound

Associated Organ: Small intestine
Element: Fire
Season: Summer
Color: Red
Negative Emotions: Impatience, hastiness, arrogance, cruelty, violence
Positive Emotions: Love, joy, honor, sincerity, happiness, creativity, enthusiasm
Sound: Haw-w-w-w-w-w (mouth wide open)
Parts of the Body: Armpits, inner arms
Sense/Body Substance: Tongue, speech, sweat

1. Position: Be aware of the heart and smile into it. Take a deep breath and assume the same position as for the liver's sound. Unlike the former exercise, however, you will lean slightly to the right to pull gently against the heart, which is just to the left of the center of your chest. Focus on your heart, and feel your tongue.

2. Sound: Open your mouth, round your lips, and slowly exhale the sound "haw-w-w-w-w-w-w" subvocally. Picture the pericardium (the sac around the heart) expelling heat, impatience, hastiness, arrogance, and cruelty.

3. Rest and concentrate: After having exhaled, smile into your heart, and picture a bright red color and the qualities of love, joy, honor, sincerity, and creativity entering your heart. Repeat the steps above 3 to 24 times. Practice more often to relieve sore throat, cold sores, swollen gums or tongue, jumpiness, moodiness, or heart disease.

☯ *Spleen's Sound*

Associated Organs: Pancreas, stomach
Element: Earth
Season: Indian summer
Color: Yellow
Negative Emotions: Worry, anxiety, pity
Positive Emotions: Fairness, openness, compassion, centering, balance
Sound: Who-o-o-o-o-o (from the throat, guttural)
Parts of the Body: Inner legs, groin, ribs
Sense/Body Substance: Taste, mouth, saliva

1. Position: Be aware of your spleen and smile into it. Take a deep breath as you place the fingers of both hands just beneath the sternum on your left side. You will press in with the fingers as you push your middle back outward.

2. Sound: Look up, and gently push your fingertips into the left of the solar plexus area, as you subvocally exhale the sound "who-o-o-o-o-o." This is more guttural, or "throaty," than the kidneys' sound, originating from the depths of the throat rather than the mouth. Feel the spleen's sound vibrate the vocal cords. Feel any worries being transformed as the virtues of fairness and honesty arise.

3. Rest and concentrate: Once you have fully exhaled, close your eyes, place your hands on your thighs, palms up, and concentrate smiling energy on your spleen, pancreas, and stomach. Breathe into these organs as you picture a bright yellow light shining in the organs. Repeat the steps above 3 to 24 times. Practice more often to eliminate indigestion, nausea, or diarrhea.

✪ Triple Heater's Sound

The triple heater (also referred to as the triple warmer) does not have the same characteristics as the other five organs as it comprises the three energy centers of the body: the upper section (brain, heart, and lungs) is hot; the middle section (liver, kidneys, stomach, pancreas, and spleen) is warm; and the lower section (large and small intestines, urinary bladder, and sexual organs) is cool. The sound "he-e-e-e-e-e" balances the temperature of the three levels by bringing hot energy down to the lower center and cold energy up to the higher centers. Specifically, hot energy from the area of the heart moves to the colder sexual region, and cold energy from the lower abdomen is moved up to the heart's region.

1. Position: Lie on your back with your arms resting palms up at your sides, and keep your eyes closed. Inhale fully into all three cavities: chest, solar plexus, and lower abdomen.

2. Sound: Exhale the sound "he-e-e-e-e-e" subvocally, flattening first your chest, then your solar plexus, and finally your lower abdomen. Imagine a large roller pressing out your breath as it moves from your head down to your sexual center.

3. Rest and concentrate: When you have fully exhaled, concentrate on your entire body. Repeat the above steps from 3 to 6 times. Practice more often to relieve insomnia or stress.

Daily Sound Practice before Bedtime

Practice the six healing sounds before going to bed at night. This will help decelerate the body, promote good sleep, and cool down any overheated organs. Before you go to sleep, clear any negative emotions so that the positive emotions can grow. Clearing out the negative emotions will chase away bad dreams and nightmares. You can sleep well and connect to the universal mind to recharge your energy.

If you have problems or feel ill, attain the sensation of emptiness and send these disturbances up into the universal mind. Trust that this force will help you. In the morning smile inwardly and see whether you can find answers to your disturbances. Often the answer will be there for you when you awake.*

---

*For more information on the Six Healing Sounds practice, see *The Six Healing Sounds* (Rochester, Vt.: Destiny Books, 2009). Included with this book is an audio CD that will allow you to hear each of the sounds.

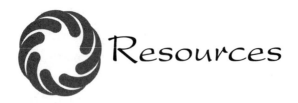 # Resources

In this section we have listed several sources for the cleansing supplements and colonic supplies that we have recommended throughout the book, as well as sources for colloidal silver, kombucha starter, revitalized water, and more information on acid and alkaline balance in the diet.

Cleansing Supplements and Colonic Supplies

V. E. Irons, Inc.

P.O. Box 34710
North Kansas City, MO 64116
Toll free: 800-544-8147
Phone: 816-221-3719
Fax: 816-221-1272
E-mail: info@veirons.com
Website: www.veirons.com

V. E. Irons is home of Vit-Ra-Tox Products and manufacturers of quality whole food supplements since 1946. We have listed several products available from V. E. Irons below, but see their website for the full product line.

Detoxificant (bentonite)

This substance is a natural and powerful detoxificant derived from bentonite, a mineral-rich volcanic clay. The active detoxifying ingredient is montmorillonite ("mont-mor-ill-o-nite"). Montmorillonite possesses the ability to absorb about 40 times its own weight in positively charged substances present in the alimentary canal. Because montmorillonite has such strong adsorptive properties and is not digested, it tightly binds material to be excreted. It is a perfect accompaniment to the Intestinal Cleanser (see below). Mixed together in juice, this cleansing drink offers the scrubbing and roughage benefits from soluble and insoluble fiber from psyllium, and the detoxification properties of bentonite.

Intestinal Cleanser (psyllium)

Intestinal Cleanser is a finely ground powder of imported psyllium husk and seed. As it contains primarily fiber and no laxative or herbal stimulants, it can be used on a daily basis to assist normal bowel peristalsis. Psyllium has a hydrophilic (water-loving) action that softens hardened mucus lining the bowel wall, facilitating its elimination. The Intestinal Cleanser and Detoxificant (see above) are ideal companion products to be used together for maximum alimentary canal detoxification.

GreenLife (chlorophyll gel capsules)

GreenLife is a 100 percent vegetable food containing 92 percent dried extracted juices of organically grown cereal grasses: barley, oats, rye, and wheat (no chemical fertilizers or insecticides are used); and 8 percent papain, beets, and sea kelp. The grasses are cut at the young, rapidly growing stage, when the maximum nutrition is in the blade. GreenLife is a concentrated product, retaining its natural balance as a complete all-food supplement. It is nontoxic in any consumable amount, and helps balance nutritional deficiencies resulting from consumption of devitalized and processed foods.

Pro-Gest (vegetarian pancreatic enzymes)

The active ingredient in Pro-Gest is papain, which is derived from the papaya fruit. Papain is a natural proteolytic enzyme that breaks down proteins and supports a healthy digestive process. Other ingredients include papaya seed meal, Russian black radish, and betaine hydrochloride in a base of dried juice from organically grown beets—the same powder used for Whole Beet Plant Juice Tablets (see below). The betaine hydrochloride acts to supplement the natural hydrochloric acid in the stomach.

Whole Beet Plant Juice Tablets

The beets used for this product are organically grown. The whole beet (leaves, stems, and root) is juiced, and the extract is vacuum dried at low temperature to retain maximum quantities of the enzymes, vitamins, and mineral factors. Unlike inorganic sources of iron, the body assimilates iron from the beetroot very easily, because iron is found in an organic complex. Beets also contain potassium, magnesium, phosphorous, calcium, sulfur, iodine, vitamins and many trace minerals.

Fasting Plus (enzyme supplement)

Never before has the use of antacids and gastric medication to treat indigestion been so prevalent. These types of drugs block the body's natural digestive processes, but our enzymatic supplement aids the digestion process by providing natural digestive enzymes to break down food and promote assimilation of nutrients. Each tablet contains two layers of digestive enzymes. The outer portion contains pepsin, which digests protein into soluble amino acids, proteases, and peptones. Pepsin is activated by the low pH of the stomach, so people suspected of gastric acid deficiency would benefit from it. The inner portion of the tablet becomes activated in the small intestine, and contains natural digestive agents: bovine bile salts that promote absorption of lipids and activate pancreatic lipase (a fat-digesting enzyme), and the pancreatic substances amylase (for starch) and proteases (for protein), plus tyrosine, chymotrypsin, and other proteolytic enzymes. Because the inner portion is intended to work in the intestine, the tablets should be swallowed whole.

Wheat Germ Oil/Flaxseed Oil

The wheat germ oil capsules contain 73 percent wheat germ oil, an excellent source of the natural vitamin E complex; and 27 percent flaxseed oil, a rich source of unsaturated, essential fatty acids including: alpha linolenic acid, omega-6, and omega-3. Vitamin E is an essential dietary component that is necessary for antioxidant activity in membranes. It regenerates other cellular antioxidants (i.e., selenium and glutathione) after they become oxidized. The essential fatty acids also must be obtained in the diet, and are precursors for many hormones and metabolically active compounds. The natural vitamin E in our foods is destroyed during cooking and processing due to heat, light, air, and freezing. Grains lose up to 80 percent of their vitamin E content when milled. Commercially processed vegetable oils are low in vitamin E. It has become quite clear that there is a need for natural vitamin E supplementation in our modern diets.

Bernard Jensen International

1255 Linda Vista Drive
San Marcos, CA 92078
Phone: 760-471-9977
Fax: 760-471-9989
E-mail: info@bernardjensen.com
Website: www.bernardjensen.com

Bernard Jensen International carries a wide variety of natural supplements and detoxifying products including colonic boards and supplies. We have listed a few of their supplements below, but see their website for the full range of products.

Vitamin C

This natural source vitamin C tablet contains natural vitamin C derived from dehydrated juice of the acerola berry and wild Spanish orange. These food sources provide the vitamin C complex (i.e., bioflavonoids and other synergistic nutrients), factors not present in supplements that use ascorbic acid (chemical form of vitamin C).

This vitamin C has a 100 mg equivalent of ascorbic acid per serving, supplying 110 percent of the Recommended Daily Allowance (RDA). Because vitamin C is constantly being utilized, it should be taken in small repeated doses throughout the day. Chewable tablets are ideal for this purpose, providing easy and rapid absorption of the natural vitamin C complex.

Nova Scotia Dulse (dulse tablets)

Nova Scotia Dulse is a sea vegetable that is a natural source of essential vitamins, ions, sea salt, and roughage. Harvested from the cold waters of the North Atlantic, this premium dulse is then sun-dried to preserve the natural nutrients. Each tablet provides you with a variety of essential vitamins, minerals, protein, and trace elements the way nature intended. These tablets give you the sodium necessary to assist in moving the waste from the cells in a cellular cleanse.

Niacin

Niacin or nicotonic acid, a water-soluble B-complex vitamin and antihyperlipidemic agent, is 3-pyridinecarboxylic acid. It is a white, crystalline powder, sparingly soluble in water. Niacin is essential in energy production at the cellular level. Niacin helps maintain proper metabolic function. Niacin is used for lowering the levels of LDL ("bad") cholesterol or of triglyceride in the blood of certain patients. It may be used in combination with diet or other medicines. It may also be used for other conditions as determined by your doctor. It works by decreasing the amount of a certain protein that is necessary for the formation of cholesterol in the body.

Colema Boards of California, Inc.

P.O. Box 1879
Cottonwood, CA 96022
Toll free: 800-745-2446
Phone: 530-347-5700
Fax: 530-347-2336

E-mail: info@colema.com

Website: www.colema.com

The best source for genuine Colema colonic boards, tubing, and supplies. This company also carries a wide variety of supplements and colonic cleansing products.

Colloidal Silver

www.silver-colloids.com

This website, written by a colloidal chemist, provides detailed, unbiased information about colloidal silver's properties, production, and safety. It also provides analyses of many of the colloidal silver products available to consumers.

Solutions I.E. Health Products

Website: www.solutionsie.com

Offers a wide range of health supplements, including colloidal silver.

Energized Water

Earth Transitions

44 Canyon Drive #3

Oceanside, CA 92054

E-mail: info@earthtransitions.com

Website: www.earthtransitions.com

Offers vortex water energizers, super ionized water concentrate, and the water egg for storing water, inspired by Viktor Schauberger.

World Living Water Systems

432 North Dollarton Hwy.

North Vancouver, BC V7G 1N1

Canada

Tel: 604-990-5462

Toll free: 888-644-7754

Fax: 604-904-7455

Website: www.alivewater.net

Offers several different models of vortex water revitalizers for small to large applications—from apartment size to industrial water treatment facilities.

Kombucha Starter

www.happyherbalist.com

Provides detailed information on brewing your own kombucha and sells mushroom starter kits.

www.organic-kombucha.com

Offers starter kits and information on brewing, storing, and using kombucha.

pH-Balanced Diet

www.thealkalinediet.org

Provides extensive information about acid/alkaline balance, food lists, and resources for further information.

www.trans4mind.com/nutrition/pH.html

Includes a how-to on urine and saliva testing, food charts, and a look at the science behind acid/alkaline food chemistry.

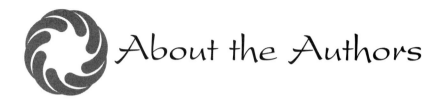# About the Authors

MANTAK CHIA

Mantak Chia has been studying the Taoist approach to life since childhood. His mastery of this ancient knowledge, enhanced by his study of other disciplines, has resulted in the development of the Universal Healing Tao system, which is now being taught throughout the world.

Mantak Chia was born in Thailand to Chinese parents in 1944. When he was six years old, he learned from Buddhist monks how to sit and "still the mind." While in grammar school he learned traditional Thai boxing, and he soon went on to acquire considerable skill in aikido, yoga, and Tai Chi. His studies of the Taoist way of life began in earnest when he was a student in Hong Kong, ultimately leading to his mastery of a wide variety of esoteric disciplines, with the guidance of several masters, including Master I Yun, Master Meugi, Master Cheng Yao Lun, and Master Pan Yu. To better understand the mechanisms behind healing energy, he also studied Western anatomy and medical sciences.

Master Chia has taught his system of healing and energizing practices to tens of thousands of students and trained more than two thousand instructors and practitioners throughout the world. He has established centers for Taoist study and training in many countries around the globe. In June of 1990, he was honored by the International Congress of Chinese Medicine and Qi Gong (Chi Kung), which named him the Qi Gong Master of the Year.

WILLIAM U. WEI

Born after World War II, growing up in the Midwest area of the United States, and trained in Catholicism, William Wei became a student of the Tao and started studying under Master Mantak Chia in the early 1980s. In the later 1980s he became a senior instructor of the Universal Healing Tao, specializing in one-on-one training. In the early 1990s William Wei moved to Tao Garden, Thailand, and assisted Master Mantak Chia in building Tao Garden Taoist Training Center. For six years William traveled to over thirty countries, teaching with Master Mantak Chia and serving as marketing and construction coordinator for the Tao Garden. Upon completion of Tao Garden in December 2000, he became project manager for all the Universal Tao Publications and products. With the purchase of a mountain with four waterfalls in southern Oregon, USA, in the late 1990s, William Wei is presently completing a Taoist Mountain Sanctuary for personal cultivation, higher-level practices, and ascension. William Wei is the coauthor with Master Chia of *Sexual Reflexology*, *Living in the Tao*, and the Taoist poetry book of 366 daily poems, *Emerald River*, which expresses the feeling, essence, and stillness of the Tao. He is also the cocreator with Master Mantak Chia of the Universal Healing Tao formula cards, Chi Cards (six sets of over 240 formulas) under the pen name The Professor—Master of Nothingness, the Myth that takes the Mystery out of Mysticism. William U. Wei, also known as Wei Tzu, is a pen name for this instructor so the instructor can remain anonymous and can continue to become a blade of grass in a field of grass.

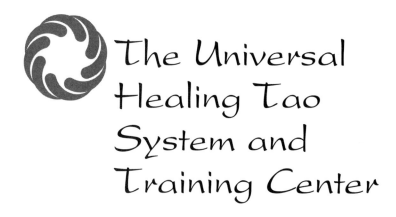

The Universal Healing Tao System and Training Center

THE UNIVERSAL HEALING TAO SYSTEM

The ultimate goal of Taoist practice is to transcend physical boundaries through the development of the soul and the spirit within the human. That is also the guiding principle behind the Universal Healing Tao, a practical system of self-development that enables individuals to complete the harmonious evolution of their physical, mental, and spiritual bodies. Through a series of ancient Chinese meditative and internal energy exercises, the practitioner learns to increase physical energy, release tension, improve health, practice self-defense, and gain the ability to heal him- or herself and others. In the process of creating a solid foundation of health and well-being in the physical body, the practitioner also creates the basis for developing his or her spiritual potential by learning to tap into the natural energies of the sun, moon, earth, stars, and other environmental forces.

The Universal Healing Tao practices are derived from ancient techniques rooted in the processes of nature. They have been gathered and integrated into a coherent, accessible system for well-being that works directly with the life force, or chi, that flows through the meridian system of the body.

Master Chia has spent years developing and perfecting techniques for teaching these traditional practices to students around the world through ongoing classes, workshops, private instruction, and healing sessions, as well as books and video and audio products. Further information can be obtained at www.universal-tao.com.

THE UNIVERSAL HEALING TAO TRAINING CENTER

The Tao Garden Resort and Training Center in northern Thailand is the home of Master Chia and serves as the worldwide headquarters for Universal Healing Tao activities. This integrated wellness, holistic health, and training center is situated on eighty acres surrounded by the beautiful Himalayan foothills near the historic walled city of Chiang Mai. The serene setting includes flower and herb gardens ideal for meditation, open-air pavilions for practicing Chi Kung, and a health and fitness spa.

The center offers classes year round, as well as summer and winter retreats. It can accommodate two hundred students, and group leasing can be arranged. For information on courses, books, products, and other Universal Tao resources, see below.

Universal Healing Tao Center

274 Moo 7, Luang Nua, Doi Saket, Chiang Mai, 50220 Thailand
Tel: (66)(53) 495-596 Fax: (66)(53) 495-852
E-mail: universaltao@universal-tao.com
Website: www.universal-tao.com

For information on retreats and the health spa, contact:

Tao Garden Health Spa and Resort

E-mail: info@tao-garden.com, taogarden@hotmail.com
Website: www.tao-garden.com

Good Chi • Good Heart • Good Intention

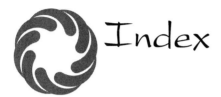

Index

Pages in *italics* refer to illustrations.

BOOKS OF RELATED INTEREST

Taoist Cosmic Healing
Chi Kung Color Healing Principles for Detoxification and
Rejuvenation
by Mantak Chia

Healing Love through the Tao
Cultivating Female Sexual Energy
by Mantak Chia

Chi Self-Massage
The Taoist Way of Rejuvenation
by Mantak Chia

Taoist Shaman
Practices from the Wheel of Life
by Mantak Chia and Kris Deva North

Living in the Tao
The Effortless Path of Self-Discovery
by Mantak Chia and William U. Wei

Healing Light of the Tao
Foundational Practices to Awaken Chi Energy
by Mantak Chia

The Healing Energy of Shared Consciousness
A Taoist Approach to Entering the Universal Mind
by Mantak Chia

The Six Healing Sounds
Taoist Techniques for Balancing Chi
by Mantak Chia

INNER TRADITIONS • BEAR & COMPANY
P.O. Box 388
Rochester, VT 05767
1-800-246-8648
www.InnerTraditions.com

Or Contact your local bookseller